ONCOLOGY
ENTRANCE EXAMINATION

**(Includes Important Text, Original
Solved MCQs and their Explanations)**

W0080810

ONCOLOGY
ENTRANCE EXAMINATION

(Includes Important Text, Original
Solved MCQs and their Explanations)

THIRD EDITION

Editors
Dr. M.S. Bhatia
MD, MNAMS, Dip. WPA
Prof. & Head, Department of Psychiatry,
University College of Medical Sciences &
Associated GTB Hospital,
Shahdara, Delhi - 110 095 (India)

&

Dr. (Mrs.) Nirmaljit Kaur
MD
Senior Specialist, Department of Microbiology,
Dr. R.M.L. Hospital,
New Delhi - 110 001 (India)

CBS

CBS Publishers & Distributors Pvt. Ltd.
New Delhi • Bengaluru • Chennai • Kochi • Kolkata • Mumbai
Hyderabad • Nagpur • Patna • Pune • Jharkhand • Uttarakhand • Dhaka

ISBN: 978-93-88902-80-9

First Edition: 2006
Reprint: 2009
Second Edition: 2014
Reprint: 2015, 2017
Third Edition: 2019

Published by **Satish Kumar Jain** and produced by **Varun Jain** for **CBS Publishers & Distributors Pvt. Ltd.,**
4819/XI Prahlad Street, 24 Ansari Road, Daryaganj, New Delhi - 110002
delhi@cbspd.com, cbspubs@airtelmail.in • www.cbspd.com
Ph.: 23289259, 23266861, 23266867 • Fax: 011-23243014

Corporate Office: 204 FIE, Industrial Area, Patparganj, Delhi - 110 092
Ph: 49344934 • Fax: 011-49344935
E-mail: publishing@cbspd.com • publicity@cbspd.com

Branches:
- *Bengaluru:* 2975, 17th Cross, K.R. Road, Bansankari 2nd Stage, Bengaluru - 70 • Ph: +91-80-26771678/79 • Fax: +91-80-26771680
  E-mail: cbsbng@gmail.com, bangalore@cbspd.com
- *Chennai:* No. 7, Subbaraya Street, Shenoy Nagar, Chennai - 600030
  Ph: +91-44-26681266, 26680620 • Fax: +91-44-42032115
  E-mail: chennai@cbspd.com
- *Kochi:* Ashana House, 39/1904, A.M. Thomas Road, Valanjambalam, Ernakulum, Kochi • Ph: +91-484-4059061-65
  Fax: +91-484-4059065 • E-mail: cochin@cbspd.com
- *Kolkata:* 6-B, Ground Floor, Rameshwar Shaw Road, Kolkata - 700014
  Ph: +91-33-22891126/7/8 • E-mail: kolkata@cbspd.com
- *Mumbai:* 83-C, Dr. E. Moses Road, Worli, Mumbai - 400018
  Ph: +91-9833017933, 022-24902340/41 • E-mail: mumbai@cbspd.com

Representatives:

• Bhubaneswar	0-9911037372	• Hyderabad	0-9885175004	• Jharkhand	0-9811541605
• Nagpur	0-9021734563	• Patna	0-9334159340	• Pune	0-9623451994
• Uttarakhand	0-9716462459	• Dhaka (Bangladesh)	01912-003485		

Printed at:
J.S. Offset Printers, Delhi (India)

Dedicated to

Respected Teachers
&
Beloved Students

PREFACE

Oncology is a rapidly advancing field. Its new allied branches are coming up. In a competitive examination, more and more emphasis is being laid on these allied disciplines. But most of the standard textbooks of genetics have failed to devote adequate space to these new disciplines.

This book has been written with the aim to outline the major areas of Oncology i.e Factual data, Commonest cause, Basic concepts and *Recent advances.* This book is not merely an addition to the existing list of books on MCQ's but a sincere ambition and an honest attempt to make it a useful and practical companion to both medical graduates and postgraduates. The present book consists of original solved MCQ's from the *Question Banks* of various important examinations (AIIMS, Delhi, PGI, All India etc.), Important text and original solved MCQ's. have also been added. We hope that this will help the candidates in performing better in the examination.

All suggestions for the modification of this book are welcome and will be duly acknowledged.

—Editors

CONTENTS

IMPORTANT TEXT OF ONCOLOGY

IMPORTANT POINTS TO REMEMBER

* Molecular policemans is Tumor suppressor gene P53

* MC tumor suppressor gene lost or mutated in human cancer is **P53**

* Most useful characteristic on pathologic diagnosis of malignancy is **lack of normal differentiation** (ANAPLASIA).

* A second malignant tumor for which a patient with retinoblastoma is most susceptibel is OSTEOSARCOMA.

* The carcinogenic effect of solar radiation is greatest in the spectral range of **290-320 nm** (UV-B radiation)

* Carcinogenic substane in tobacco smoke is **TAR.**

* MC malignancy found in increased incidence in patient treated wtih Alkylating agent is **AML.**

* MC malignancy found in increased incidene is receipient of organ transplants, who are treated with immunosuppressive agent is **Histocytic Lymphoma**

* Anticancer vitamins = A, E & C.

* Cofactor in development of African Burkitt's Lymphoma is **Holoendemic Malaria.**

* The tumor marker of greatest use to the clinician is **HCG.**

* The principal means of staging many neoplastic diseases is **surgery.**

* Target for radiation induced cell death is **DNA.**

* Time period within which cellular repair is normally complete after radiation exposure is **4 to 6 hour.**

* Best treatment for an impending spinal cord compression in a patient with metastatic carcinoma is RADIOTHERAPY.

* Most radiosensitive tissues in body is **Bone marrow** and **Gonads.**

* Treatment of choice for disseminated malignant disease is **systemic chemotherapy.**

* Neoadjuvant refers to administration of chemotherapy prior to surgery.

* A partial response to therapy is a **50%** decrease in the product of the greatest perpendicular diameter of one or more lesions.

* **Progressive disease** means :
  1. At least **25% increase** in the product of the greatest perpendicular diameter of one lesions.
  2. The appearance of **new lesions.**
* Classic **S-phase** specific agent is Cytarabine.
* **M-Phase** specific agent is Vincristine, vinblastin.
* Anticancer drug which is **severe vesicants** are :
  1. Doxorubicin
  2. Daunorubicin
  3. Mitomycin-C
  4. Nitrogen mustard.
* The **MC** dose-limiting toxicity of ankylating agents is myelosuppression.
* Anticancer drug having disulfiram like effect is **Procarbazine.**
* MAO inhibitor used as anticancer drug is **Procarbazine.**
* Carcinogenic anticancer drugs are Procarabzine, alkylating agents.
* Anticancer drug which has **maximum emetogenic** potential is Cisplatin.
* Most effective antiemetic agent used in cancer chemotherapy is Ondansetron.
* Anticancer drugs causing Alopecia (DDVCP)
  → Dactinomycin
  → Doxorubicin
  → Vincristine
  → Cyclophosphamide
  → Pacitaxel (Taxil
* **Chemosensitizing Agents** (agents which reverses P-glycoprotein mediated multidrug resistance) includes.
  → Verapamil
  → Quinine
  → Cyclosporin - A.
  → Buthionine Sulfoximine (deplets glutathion levels)
* Clincal Trials used to accept a new anticancer drug in clinical use consists of :
  a. **Phase I**-trials are performed to determine **drug toxicity** in humans.
  b. **Phase II**-trials are designed to determine if a drug has activity in a particular tumor type.
  c. **Phase III**-->trials are designed to test an agent against the standard existing therapy for a particular tumor.

Endocrine therapy of malignancy

	Hormone/drug used		Tumor susceptible

a. **Adrenal steroids :**
   - Prednisolone — 1. Lymphatic leukemias
   - Methylprednisolone — 2. Lymphoma
   - Dexemathasone — 3. Breast carcinoma

b. **Androgens :**
   - Fluxoxymesterone → Breast carcinomas

c. **Antiandrogens :**
   - Flutamide, Cyproteron → Disseminated Prostate carcinoma

d. **Estrogens :**
   - Diethylstibesterol (DES) — 1. Disseminated prostate carcinoma
   - Ethinyl estradiol — 2. Breast carcinoma

e. **Antiestrogens :**
   - Tamoxifen → Breast carcinoma

f. **Progestins :**
   - Medroxyprogesterone — 1. Endometrial carcinoma
   - Megestrol acetate — 2. Breast carcinoma

g. **Aromatase inhibitor :**
   - Aminoglutethimide — 1. Metastatic breast carcinomas
   - — 2. Disseminated prostate carcinoma

h. **GnRH agonist :**
   - Leuprolide → Disseminated prostate carcinoma
   - Buserelin

i. **Somatostatin analogues :**
   - Octreotide — 1. Metastatic carcinoid tumors
   - — 2. VIP secreting tumors,

Biological Therapy

Agent used   Malignancy

a.   Recombinant interferon →
   - (i) Hairy cell leukemia
   - (ii) AIDS-related Kaposi's sarcoma
   - (iii) Stable phase CML
   - (iv) Low grade NHL
   - (v) Multiple myeloma
   - (vi) Melanoma
   - (vii) Renal cell carcinoma
   - (viii) Ovarian carcinoma

b.   Recombinant inteleukin-2->   (i)   Metastatic melanoma
                                    (ii)   Renal cell carcinoma
                                    (iii) Ovarian carcinoma
c.   Corynebacterium parvum   Ovarian carcinoma
d.   BCG   (i)   CA-in-situ of urinary bladder
                                    (ii)   Malignant melanoma
e.   Levamisol   Dukes-C adenocarcinoma of colon.

Pathological findings in biopsies from patients with metastatic cancer of unknown primary site :

Findings	Suggested primary site
Psammoma bodies	→ (i) Ovarian carcinomas
	(ii) Papillary CA of thyroid
	(iii) Transitional Meningioma
Signet ring cells	→ CA stomach
Thyroglobulin	→ Thyroid malignancy
Leukocyte common antgen (LCA)	→ Lymphoid neoplasm
Calcitonin	→ Medullary Ca. Thyroid
Leu-M1	→ Hodgkins disease
Myoglobin	→ Rhabdomyosarcoma
HMB 45	→ Melanoma
Actin-myosin filament	→ Rhabdomyosarcoma
Desmin	→ Sarcoma
Oestrogen and Progesterone receptor	→ Breast CA
S-100	→ Neuroendocrine tumors
PSA/PAP	→ Prostate carcinoma
Secretory granules	→ Neuroendocrine tumors
Premelanosomes	→ Melanoma
Placental alkaline Phosphatase	→ Germ cell neoplasm

Biopsy findings in carcinoma

(i)   Epithelial membrane antigen
(ii)   Cytokeratin intermediate filaments
(iii)   CEA
(iv)   Desomosomes
(v)   Vimentin

Cytogenetic marker of malignancy

t (11; 22)	(i) Ewings' sarcoma
	(ii) Primitive neuroectodermal tumor
t (8; 14)	(i) Burkitt's lymphoma
	(ii) ALL-L3
t(12; 16)	Clear cell sarcoma (melanoma of soft part)
t (2;13)	Alveolar rhabdomyosarcoma
t(x; 18	Synovial sarcoma
3p (-)	(i) Small cell CA lung
(ii)	Renal cell CA
(iii)	Mesothelioma
Isochromosome	Germ cell tumor
12p; 12q (-)	

"All purpose regimens"

In cancer chemotherapy :

(a) FAM   5-fluorouracil
                 Adriamycin (doxorubicin)
                 Mitamycin-C.

(b) FACP   5-fluorouracil
                 Adriamycin (Doxorubicin)
                 Cyclophosphamide
                 Cisplatin

* Anticancer drug causing Hemolytic-Uremic syndrome = Mitomycin-C.
* Anticancer drugs inhibiting the enzyme topoisomerase I is
  (i) Irinotecan
  (II) Topotecan

Anticancer drugs inhibiting the enzyme topoisomerase II is
  (i) Doxorubicin
  (ii) Daunorubicin
  (iii) Etoposide
  (iv) Teniposide

* Tumors most frequently associated with clinically recognised ectopic hromone production are :
  1. Small cell CA lung   2.   Carcinoids
  3. Pancreatic islet tumors
  4. Squamous type of bronchogenic carcinoma of lung.

* Only class of hormone that are secreted ectopically - Peptides/Proteins
* Most frequently encountered syndromes of ectopic hormone production by malignant tumors are -

1. ACTH hypersecretion
2. Hypercalcemia
3. Organic hypoglycemia

Ectopic hormones produced by tumors

Hormones ↑	Tumors ↑
ACTH	
MSH	
Vsopressin	
Oxytocin	
Neurophysin	
CRH (Corticotropin releasing hormone)	Small cell CA of lung
Somatostatin	
Calcitonin	
Gastrin	
VIP	
Placental lactogen	
GHRH	
Gastrin releasing polypeptide	Carcinoids
Growth hormone	Large cell CA lung
Parathyroid hormone related protein	Renal cell CA
	Squamous cell CA lung
1.25 (OH)2 VitD	Lymphoma
Parthyroid hormone	Ovarian carcinoma
Parathyroid hormone	Ovarian carcinoma
Erythropoietin	Cerebellar hemangioblastoma, renal cell CA

* MC tumor responsible for **paraneoplastic syndrome** is small cell CA lung.
* Anti-HU antibody is found in paraneplastic encephalomyelitis.
* Antigen **recoverin** is responsible for cancer associated retinopathy (a paraneoplastic syndrome due to small cell lung CA).

* The Opsoclonus-Myoclonus is a PNS associated with Breast cancer in female, Medulloblastoma in child & Bronchial CA in Adult male.
* PNS associated with Non-Hodgkins lymphoma = Subacute motor neuropathy
* PNS associated with Non-Hodgkins lymphoma=Acute Demylinating neuritis (Gullian Barre Syndrome)
* PNS associated with Thymom = Myesthenia gravis
* PNS associated with Neuroblastoma - Dancing eye, dancing feet syndrome
* Most common paraneoplastic neuropathy = Sensori motor neuropathy.
* The primary target of chemotherapeutic drugs is tumor stem cells.
* Most frequently used & most successful single method of cancer therapy currently available is surgery.

Tumor Suppressor gene loss in human cancer

Tumor suppressor gene or chromosome	Neoplasm
Chromosome 1	Neuroblastoma
Chromosome 3	Lung & Renal cell CA
Chromosome 5	Colon CA
Chromosome 11	Wilm's tumor, hepatoblas-toma, ad renal carcinoma, rhabdomyosar-coma, bladder & breast CA.
Chromosome 13 (Rb)	Retinoblastoma, Osteosarcoma, Breast, bladder & small cell lung CA
Chromosome 17 (p53)	Lung & colon CA
Chromosome 18	Colon CA
Chromosome 22	Acoustic neuroma, meningioma.

Cell cycle

* **M phase (Mitotic phase)** -It is the phase of cell division
* **G1 phase (Postmitotic phase)** - is a period fo variable duration when cellular activities and protein & RNA synthesis continue.
* **S phase (DNA synthetic phase)** -is the period in which new DNA replication occurs.
* **G2 phase (Postsynthetic phase)**-is the period in which the cell has a diploid number of chromosomes & twice the DNa content of the normal cell.

* **G0 phase (Resting phase)-**is the time during which cells donot divide.
* **Generation time ;** is the duratio of the cycle from M-phase to the next M-phase .
* **Growth Fraction :** is the number of cells in tumor mass that are actively undergoing cell division.

Cell cycle - Specificity of anticancer drugs

Classification	**Examples**
* Cellcycle specific, proliferation dependent	Hydroxyurea, Cytocin-Arabinoside
* Cell cyclesepcific, less prolife ration dependent	5-FU methotrexate
* Cell Cycle non specific, prolife. ration dependent	Cyclophosphamide, Actinomycin D. Cisplatin
* Cell cycle non-specific, prolife-ration dependent	Ntrogen mustard.

Site of action in the cell cycle

Protion of cell cycle	**Drugs**
G1 Actinomycin-D	
Early-S	Hydroxyurea cytosine-Arabinoside, 5-FU, methotrexate
Late-S	Adriamycin, Daunomycin
G2	Bleomycin, Radiation, Ectoposide, Teniposide
M	Vincristine, Vinblastin

* Chemotherapeutic agents appear to work by **First order kinetics** i.e. they kill aconstant fraction of cells rather than a constant number.
* **Dose intensity** = Drugs (mg)/surface Area (m2)/Time (week).
* **Drug Effect**=Drug conct. x Duration of exposure = C x T.
* **Sanctuary sites :** areas where the tumor is inaccessible to anticancer drugs and drug concentration over time is insufficient for cell kill. **Example** -CSF, Areas of large tumor masses with central tumor necrosis & low O2 tension.

Mechanism of resistance to anticancer drugs

	Mechanism	Example Drugs
1.	Insufficient activation of drug	Intraperitoneal cyciophosphamide, 6-mercaptopurine, 5-FU.
2.	Insufficient drug intake or defective drug transport	Methotrexate, Daunomycin
3.	Increased activation	Cytosine arabinoside
4.	Increased utilization of an alternative biochemical path way (salvage)	Cytosine-arabinoside, 5-FR
5.	Increased conc. of the target enzyme	Methotrexate
6.	Decreased requirement for a specific metabolite product	L-asparaginase
7.	Rapid DNA repair of a drug related lesion	Alkylating agent, cisplatin, carboblatin
8.	Gene amplification	Methotrexate.

SKIN -

BASAL CELL CARCINOMA

* Most common Skin cancer is **Basal cell carcinoma** (BCC)
* MC site of Basal cell CA is **Face**
* MC type of BCC is Noduloulcerative or Nodulocystic type.
* Most aggressive type of BCC is **Morphea form** (fibrosing) type.
* Type of BCC most likely to recur is **Morphea form** type.
* MC site of BCC on face is aroung the **inner canthus of** eye.
* MC sites :   (a) In male = Back (upper)
               (b) In female = (1) Lower limb (2) Back
* Type of melanoma, most frequently arising in dysplastic nevi, -superficial spreading melanoma.
* MC type of Malignant melanoma is **superficial spreading** type
* MC type of Malignant melanoma in dark-skinned people is **Acral lentiginous type.**
* Least common type of malignant melanoma in general is **Acral lentiginous type.**

* Most malignant type of M. melanoma is **Nodular type.**
* Least malignant type of M. melanoma is **Lentigo maligna type.**
* Best prognosis in **Lentigo malignant** type.
* Worst prognosis in **Amelanotic** type.
* Most important factor for prognosis in M. melanoma is STAGE at the time of presentation.
* Best single index which indicate the likelihood of metastasis in M. melanoma is Thickness of tumor.

Other Prognostic factors

* People with lesions of the extremities do better than people with melanomas of the trunk or face.
* Presence of ulceration in a lesion carries a worse prognosis.
* A large inflammatony infiltrate seen on histologic examination of a lesion is a good prognostic sign.
* **Females have a higher survival rate than males.**
* Nodular melanomas have the same prognosis as Superficial spreading type when lesions are matched for depth of invasion.

Miscellaneous point about Tumors of Skin

* MC chemical carcinogen responsible for skin cancer is arsenic.
* **Capillary leak syndrome** is due to toxicity of interleukin-2 therapy in case of M. melanoma.
* The frequency of skin cancer is proportional to the **Duration** of immunosuppression and the **extent** of sun exposure.
* **Retinoid** is used for chemoprophylaxis in multiple skin cancers.
* Unfavourable sites for M. melanoma :- scalp, hand, feet * mucous membrane.
* Gall bladder is also a site for M. melanoma.
* Skin Cancer is commoner in following situations :
  (i)   Marjolin's ulcer (burn scar)
  (ii) Repeated sloughing of skin from bullous diseases   Sq. cell
  (iii) Decubitus ulcer   CA
  (iv) Karro Cancer
  (v)   Organ transplantation
  (vi) Pt. having chronic immunosuppressive therapy

* MC site of distant metastasis is brain.
* MC site for earliest metastasis in M. melanoma is **Regional lymph node.**
* Sq. cell CA is more common on **lower lip** than upper lip.
* Shave biopsy or Curretage of a suspected melanoma is Contraindicated.
* **Pathologic conditions associated with skin malignancy :**
    * Basal cell nervus Syndrome
    * Nevus sebaceus of Jadassohn   Basal cell CA
    * Familial dysplastic nevus syndrome   Malignant melanoma
* Xeroderma pigmentosum
* Epidermodysplasia verruciformis   SQ. Cell CA.
* Epidermolysis bullosus
* Lupus erythmatosus
* MC subcutaneous neoplasm is **Lipoma**
* MC site of lipoms is **trunk.**

OSTEOLOGY

BENIGN TUMORS

* MC benign tumor if bone is **Osteochondroma**
* All benign bone tumors are painless except **Osteoid osteoma.**
* MC site for Ivory osteoma (compact osteoma) is **outer table of skull.**
* MC site for osteoid osteoma is **cortex** of long bones (Femur or Tibia).
* Osteoid osteoma can occur in any bone except skull.
* MC presenting symptoms of osteoid osteoma is PAIN
* MC **D/D** of osteoid osteoma is **Brodies abscess.**
* Osteochondroma is most common in males.
* **Mushroom like** bone tumor in X-ray -Osteochondroma.
* FAN Sign in X-ray is **diagnostic** in llier's disease (Multiple enchondromatosis).
* Maffucci's Syndrome consists of Multiple enchondroma Plus hemangioma Plus phleboliths.
* MC destructive bone tumor occurring in hand is **Enchondroma.**
* **Codman's Tumor is benign chondroblastoma**
* Chicken wire **calcification** is seen in Benign chondroblastoma
* Only **benign** tumor that metastesize to lungs is Benign chondroblastoma.
* MC site for chondromyxoid fibroma is **Tibia.**
* Bone neoplasms are classified by the Matrix produced by tumor cells.

* If osteoid osteoma is > **1 cm.** it is known as Osteoblastoma.
* Bony stalk with a cartilaginous cap in X-ray is found in **osteochondroma.**
* MC sites of chondroma are Metacarpals, Metatarsals & Phalanges.
* Benign bone tumors arising from Epiphysis :-
    * Osteochondroma
    * Benign chondroblastoma.

MALIGNANT BONE TUMORS

* MC malignant bone tumor is Secondaries in bone.
* MC primary malignant bone tumor is **Multiple myeloma.**
* MC primary malignant tumor of **long bones** is Osteogenic sarcoma.
* MC site of osteosarcoma is **lower end of femur.**
* MC type of osteosarcoma is Primary Medulary Type.
* MC presenting feature of osteosarcoma is Pain.
* MC site of metastasis in osteosarcoma is Lungs.
* Stanford's Cade's regimen is used in Tt. of osteosarcoma
* Radiological appearance in osteosarcoma.
    (i) **Codman's triangle**
    (ii) Sunray spicules
    (iii) LEG of Mutton appearance.
    (iv) Pathological fracture
    (v) Secondaries in lungs
* MC sit for chondrosarcoma if it occurs in long bones is femur.
* MC presenting feature of chondrosarcoma is mass.
* MC site of metastasis in chondrosacoma is lung
* Fluffy calcification in X-ray is seen in chondrosarcoma.
* Primary bone malignancy which is **most difficult to diagnose** even by open biopsy is chondrosarcoma.
* Surgery is the TOC in chondrosarcoma (Radioresistant).
* Osteoclastoma (Giant cell tumor) is more common in female.
* MC site of osteoclastoma is **lower end of femur.**
* MC site of metastasis in osteoclastoma is **lung.**
* **Eggshell crackling** on palpation is seen in osteoclastoma.
* MC D/D of osteoclastoma is Brown Tumor of hyperparathyroidism.
* **X-ray features** of osteoclastoma :

(i) Expand **transversely** in the bone

(ii) Sharp edges

(iii) Soap Bubble appearance.

* Ideal treatment for a gaint cell tumor of lateral condyle of lower end of femur is Radical Excision + IM fixation + turngrafting.

* Joint space is Normal in synovial sarcoma.

* Snow Storm appearance in X-ray is seen in synovial sarcoma.

* Presence of Foam cell is diagnostic in **Synovial Sarcoma.**

* MC bone tumor in children is **Ewing's tumor.**

* Most mal:gnant bone tumor in childhood is **Ewing's tumor.**

* MC site of Ewing's tumor is TIBIA

* Malignant Endothelioma=Ewing's tumor

* MC presenting symptoms in Ewing's tumor is **painful hot swelling.**

* Mc **D/D** of Ewing's tumor **is Acute osteomylitis.**

* PAS positive material found in Ewing's tumour is Glycogen

* Onion Peel apperance in X-ray is seen in **Ewing's tumor.**

* **Most radiosensitive** bone tumor is Ewing's tumor

* Pathognomonic feature of Ewing's tumor -Tumor melts by radiotherapy like snow.

* MC site of multiple myeloma is **Vertebra.**

* Sieve Skull in X-ray is seen in Multiple myeloma.

* Ossophile Tumors are primary tumors giving rise to secondaries in bone.

* MC primary tumor giving rise to secondaries in bone :

Breast   -   in female

Prostate -   in male

* MC sites of secondary bone tumor is **Vertebra**

* MC presenting features of secondary bone tumor is Pain.

* MC bone involved in metastasis from prostatic carcinoma is pelvis.

* In case of secondaries in bone **50%** of medulla is destroyed before a lesion is seen on X-ray.

* 99Tc is most valuable in indicating spread of metastasis.

* TOC for metastatic bone tumor is radiotherapy.

* MC primary tumor which gives rise ot solitary metastatic bone lesion is renal cell carcinoma.

* Physaliform cells is diagnostic in chordoma.

* MC site of Admantinoma is **Mandible.**

* MC large bone affected in Admantinoma is TIBIA.

* Admantinoma may disseminate to Inguinal Lymph Nodes.
* **Disappearing bone disease** = Hemangioma of bone
* **Phantom bone tumor** =Hamartoma.
* Storifrom arrangement of fibroblastic cells are seen in Histiocytoma.
* **Commonest site** of glomus tumor is **Phalanges.**
* Drug of choice in hypercalcemia due to bony metastesis is Mithramycin.
* Non-union after osteotomy is mostly seen with **Neurofibromatosis.**
* MC histological feature of Codman's tumor is Calcification.
* Rosette formation is characteristic of **Neuroblastoma**
* Most of the secondary tumors of bone are **Osteolytic.**
* Primary tumors that produce Osteoblastic (osteosclerotic) secondaries in the bone are **CA Prostate & Breast.**
* Diaphyseal Bone Tumors are :
    1. Ewing's tumor   2.   Admantinoma
    3. Enchondroma   4.   Secondaries
    5. M. myeloma.
* Epiphyseal Bone Tumors are :
    1. Osteoclastoma   2.   Codman's tumor 3. Osteochondroma
* Metaphyseal Bone Tumor is **Osteogenic Sarcoma**

HEAD & NECK

* MC location for a mucous cyst or **mucocele** is labial mucosa of lower lip.
* MC salivary gland which gives rise to a **Ranula** is the sublingual S. Gland.
* MC site for **Peripheral giant cell reparative granuloma** is Gingiva.
* MC site for **papillomas** are Tongue & Larynx.
* MC site for **Granular cell myoblastoma** is larynx.
* Granular cell myoblastoma is derived from Schwann cells.
* MC ulcer of oral cavity is Idiopathic Aphthous Ulcer.
* MC site for **Nectrotizing sialometaplasia** is Hard Palate.
* MC bone of head & neck region, involved by **fibrous dysplasia** is mandible or Maxilla.
* MC gene (oncogene) associated with sq. cell. CA of head & neck is **INT-2 gene.**

Etiology & Risk factors :

* Tobacco
* Betal nut   Oral cavity & lip
* UV radiation-(CA.Lip)
* Alcohol
* Poor oral hygiene
* Smoking
* Sepsis
* Sharp edge of tooth
* Syphilis
* Spices
* HPV type 16-Sq. cell. CA of larynx, buccal mucosa, tongue.
* HPV type 16 & 18-**Nasal cavity & paranasal sinuses.**
* EBV-**Nasopharyngeal CA.**
* Wood workers   Adenocarcinoma of nasal
* Workers in shoe industry   cavity & paranasal sinuses.
* Radiation therapy
* Plumme-vinson syndrome-   **Post cricoid** CA of hypopharynx.
* AIDS   Sq. cell. CA of upper
                             aerodigestive tract.
* Barrett's esophagus and esophagitis   Advanced **laryngeal** CA.
* Familial
* **Visualization** of the entire upper aerodigestive tract is the sin qua non of diagnosis.
* Recently, Leukoplakia (**White patch**) is **not** considered as premalignant itself, but simply as a evidence of chronic irritation.
* The changes from hyperplasia to dysplasia is thought to be **irreversible and the initial step** in ultimate carcinogenesis.
* Erythroplasia or Erythroplakia (**Red patch**) are premalignnat lesions and may also indicate the presence of another **adjacent malignancy.**
* **Field cancerization or condemned mucosa phenomenon** is the finding of epithelial abnormalities throughout the entire upper aerodi-gestivetract in a patient with sq. cell. CA **at one site.**
* Erythroplakia in the oral cavity increases the risk of invasive carcinoma in,
  * pharynx
  * larynx
  * esophagus
  * lung.

* Presence of synchronous malignancy (second primary tumor) is also a important feature of cancer of head & neck.
* For mucosal lesions, Pinch or Punch Biopsy is obtained at the margin away from the areas of obvious necrosis.
* Exception is the small lesion that would be completely removed by a biopsy
* MC site of distant metastasis of head & neck tumor, is lung (other sites are bone, skin & liver).
* Most common anatomic complications after surgery are nerve injuries.
* MC nerve injured after neck surgery is accessory nerves (paralysis of trapezius).
* The most appropriate approach to complication is prevention.

Staging :

* Most important (main) parameter determining the staging is size of the primary tumors.

ORAL CAVITY

A.   Carcinoma lip

* MC type is SQ. cell carcinoma
* MC site for sq. cell CA is lower lip.
* MC site for **Basal cell carcinoma** is the upper lip.
* MC sq. cell CA lip is **well differentiated stage I lesion.**
* MC bone involved by direct invasion of Ca buccal mucosa is mandible.

Hard Palate

* MC cancer of hard palate in India is epidermoid carcinoma
* MC site for tumors (both benign & malignant) of the minor salivary gland is **Hard palate.**

Oral Tongue

* Also called mobile tongue.
* Second MC site of oral cancer (after lip).
* MC cancer is Sq. cell carcinoma.
* Mc associated factors are Tobacco & Alcohol
* MC clinical type is ulcerative type.
* MC age of involvement is 6-70 years
* MC site of involvement is mid portion of lateral margin.
* MC precancerous lesion in **India** is submucosal fibrosis.
* MC route of spread of lymphatic
* MC mode of lymphatic spread is by embolisation.

Cheek

* MC cancer cheek is Sq. cell carcinoma
* Predisposing factors are :
  * Betal nuts
  * Smoking
  * Alcohol
  * Candida infection
  * Submucous fibrosis
* MC clinical type of Ca cheek is papilliferous growth.

PHARYNX

Nasopharynx

* **"Frog-face appearance"** in Nasopharyngeal angiofibroma is due to extension of the tumor laterally.
* Method of choice to differentiate angiofibroma from a adenoid is angiography.
* MC type of Ca nasopharynx is non-keratinizing Sq. cell carcinoma.
* MC site of origin is the fossa of rosenmuller (**or, Posterior superior wall).**
* MC symptoms is nasal stuffiness or obstruction.
* MC cranial nerve involved in infiltration due to nasopharyngeal carcinoma is abducent (followed by Trigeminal & occulomotor).
* MC **sign** is a mass in the neck, secondary to cervical metastases.
* Nasopharyngeal Sq. cell CA having **best prognosis** is the mixed non-keratinizing type.
* Nasopharyngeal Sq. cell CA having **worst prognosis** is keratinizing type.
* **Association** of nasopharyngeal CA :
  * Genetic susceptibility (located on **HLA-A2** locus)
  * Infection by **Epstein-Barr Virus** (IgA antibody assay is useful).
  * Ingestion of **salted fish** (in China)
* Keystone of the investigation of Ca nasopharynx is radiography.
* **Esthesioneuroblastomas :** are malignant tumor of nasopharynx, arises from olfactory epithelium connected to the cribriform plate of ethmoid bone.
  It readily invades the ethmoid sinuses and may involve the orbit.
* MC cancer of oropharynx is Sq. cell carcinoma.

* MC site is lateral wall
* MC clinical type of oropharyngeal cancer is ulcerative type

Hypopharynx

* MC cancer is Sq. cell carcinoma (Ulcerative type).
* MC site of pyriform sinus.
* MC symptoms are Pain & dysphagia.
* There is submucosal extension of tumor of hypopharynx

Benign tumors

* MC benign tumor of nose & paranasal sinuses are inverted papilloma (also called as Schneiderian Papilloma, Squamous or, Papillomatosis).
* Inverted papilloma arises **exclusively** from the lateral nasal wall.
* Inverted papilloma can be associated with concurrent and subsequent invasive sq. cell carcinoma.
* Surface of the inverted papilloma is covered with Transitional Epithelium (alternate layer of squamous & columnar epithelium).
* TOC in inverted papilloma is wide local excision.
* MC symptoms produced by inverted papilloma is Nasal obstruction.
* MC site of osteoma is frontal sinus.

Carcinoma of nose & paramasal sinus

* MC type is Sq. cell carcinoma.
* MC site of origin is **Maxillary antrum.**
* Second MC type of cancer is Adenocystic carcinoma (also called cylindroma).
* MC symptoms is Nasal obstruction (for cancers of **Ethmoid** sinus) Facial or dental pain (for CA, of **Maxillary** sinus).

TUMORS OF LARYNX

Benign tumors

* MC benign tumor of larynx is papilloma
* MC site is true vocal cord.
* MC symptoms is hoarseness
* MC presentation is pedunculated exophytic mass.
* TOC of papilloma larynx is laser obliteration.
* MC site for both Oncocytoma and Granular cell myoblastoma is true vocal cord.
* MC site of chondromas of larynx is cricoid cartilage
* TOC in laryngeal paraganglioma is partial laryngectomy.

Carcinoma of larynx

* MC malignancy of the upper aerodigestive tract. (second MC site is tonsil.

* MC cancer of larynx is Sq. cell carcinoma

* MC site is **Glottic** (true vocal cord)

* MC & Earliest symptom is hoarseness of voice.

* MC predisposing factor is tobacco (smoking).

* Glotic cancer is common in **male,** while supraglottic cancer is common in **female.**

* Cervical lymphnode metastasis is commonest in **Transglottic cancers** (involving the glottis, supraglottis & subglottis).

* Second common cancer having lymph node metastasis is **supraglottic cancers.**

8 Thyroid gland trachea and strap muscles of the neck is commonly involved in **Subglottic cancers.**

* MC laryngeal cacncer associated with **Respiratory obstruction and a Normal voice** is subglottic.

* TOC in **Early** Glottic cancer is radiotherapy.

* TOC in **Advanced** Glottic cancer is vertical hemilaryngectomy.

* TOC in **Transglottic cancer is** total laryngectomy.

* TOC in Glottic cancer which **crosses** the anterior or posterior commissure is total laryngectomy.

* Most reliable predictor of local control in laryngeal cancer is free margin status.

* TOC of **supraglottic** cancer is supraglottic (horizontal) laryngectomy with pre or postoperative radiotherapy.

* Toc in **subglottic** cancer is combined surgery & radiotherapy. (Initial therapy->Radiotherapy, For recurrence -> Surgery in form of total laryngectomy and removal of paratracheal lymph nodes).

* TOC of carcinoma-in-situ of larynx is stripping of vocal cord.

* Toc in **carcinoma of larynx with stridor** is tracheostomy.

* CA larynx having best prognosis is **Glottic cancer.**

Salivary Glands

* MC benign tumor of salivary gland is pleomorphic adenoma (mixed tumor).

* MC site of tumors of salivary gland is parotid gland.

* MC cause of solitary mass in salivary gland is Pleomorphic Adenoma.
* MC presentation of pleomorphic odenoma is solitary mass.
* MC malignancy arise from previous pleomorphic adenoma is adenocarcinoma.
* Danger to facial nerve injury is more in removal of recurrent pleomorphic adenoma than primary one.
* MC oncocytoma is common in minor salivary glands
* MC presentation is lump in nasopharynx & larynx.
* MC cancer of parotid gland is mucoepidermoid carcinoma.
* MC cancer of submandibular gland and Minor salivary glands is adenoid cystic carcinoma.
* MC site of Minor salivary gland cancer is **Hard palate.**
* MC site of Adenoid cystic carcinoma is minor salivary glands
* MC site of acinic cell carcinoma is parotid gland (**almost exclusively**).
* MC carcinoma of salivary glands having a great propencity for local recurrence and perineural invasion is adenoid cystic carcinoma.
* MC cancer arising from previous pleomorphic adenoma is adenocarcinoma.
* MC salivary gland involved by carcinoma-ex-pleomorphic adenoma is parotid.
* Least common cancer of salivary gland is primary Sq. cell carcinoma.
* Cribriform or, lace like appearance of myoepithelial cells is a feature of adenoid cystic carcinoma.
* **MC symptom** of salivary gland cancer is pain.
* MC presentation of salivary gland cancer is discrete mass.
* MC salivary gland tumor of childhood is mucoepidermoid tumor
* MC site of distant metastasis in cancers of salivary gland is **Lung.**
* Most specific sign of salivary gland malignancy, even without the presence of discrete mass in peripheral nerve palsy.
* Salivary gland cancers having **best prognosis** is acinic cell carcinoma.
* The incidence of malignancy among salivary gland tumors varies inversly with the size of the gland.
* MC salivary gland for which prophylactic neck dissection is done as treatment of cancer is submandibular gland.
* Least time interval, which must be lapsed before a pleomorphic adenoma turn into malignant tumor is 10 years.
* Confirmatory method of diagnosis of salivary gland cancer is frozen section examination.

* For parotid tumor, needle biopsy for diagnosis may be done by peroral route.
* Radical surgery in presence of distant-metastases is **contraindicated** in all types of cancers of salivary gland except Adenoid cystic carcinoma.
* MC graft used for reconstruction of facial nerve repair is sural nerve graft.
* When the facial nerve must be divided, it should be repaired (if functioning) prior to surgery.
* Time taken for complete recovery of nerve grafting may be from **18 months to 2 years** 1.5-2 yr)

EAR

* Glomus Tympanicum is the tumor of **Tympanic plexus.**
* Earliest symptoms of a glomus tumor is **Pulsatile Tinnitus.**
* Brown's sign (pulsation of the tympanic membrane that is inhibited by positive pressure applied to the tympanic membrane by a pneumatic otoscope) is present in tumors of middle ear.

JAW

* MC site of **Paget's disease of jaw** is maxilla.
* Multiple ostiomas of the mandible (particularly at the **angle**) is a feature of gardners syndrome.
* MC malignant tumor of **mandible** is Sq. cell carcinoma.
* TOC in CA of mandible is surgical resection (usually, **Segmental resection).**

Miscellaneous points about

HEAD & NECK TUMORS

* MC neoplasm of Head & neck in children is **Lymphoma.**
* Second MC head & neck tumor in children is rhabdomyosarcoma.
* MC cancer of paranasal sinus following long term exposure to wood dust is adenocarcinoma.
* MC cancer of paranasal sinus after radiation therapy for bilateral retinoblastoma is adenocarcinoma.
* "ANDY GUMP DEFORMITY" is due to destruction of the contour of the chin after removal of anterior part of the mandibular arch.
* MC primary cancer (**outside the head & neck**) which gives metastases to neck is lung cancer.
* MC type of soft-tissue sarcoma in adult is malignant fibrous histiocytoma.
* Mc type of soft-tissue sarcoma in **children is Rhabdomyosarcoma.**

* MC site of metastasis from Esthesioneuroblastoma is cervical lymph nodes.
* MC paragnaglioma is the carotid body tumor.
* Mc manifestation fo the treatment failure in case of malignant fibrous histiocytoma is local recurrence.
* MC source of bleeding in case of juvenile angiofibroma is internal maxillary artery.
* Mc site of primary cancer in the head & neck which gives rise to cervical lymph node metastasis is nasopharynx. (Second MC site is **Base of tongue**).
* Composite resection is the operation for the removal of an oral tumor which includes, **Segmental resection of the mandible** and a **neck dissection.**

NERVOUS SYSTEM

TUMORS OF NERVOUS SYSTEM

* MC tumor of CNS is glioma (Second MC is econdaries).
* MC primary tumor of Brain in adult is glioblastoma multiformis (malignant Astrocytoma or, Astocytoma grade 3 or 4).
* MC solid tumor in children is brain tumor.
* MC brain tumor in children less than 7 yrs. of age is medulloblastoma.
* MC infratentorial (posterior fossa) brain tumor in children is cerebellarastrocytoma.
* MC supratentorial brain tumor in children is craniopharyngioma.
* MC primary, which gives rise to secondaries in the brain is
    * Lung cancer in Men.
    * Breast cancer in Women.
* MC tumor which have the **highest likelihood** of spread to the CNS is Malignant melanoma.
* MC route of spread by which secondaries reach the CNS is hematogenous.
* MC site of glioblastoma
    * In Adult ->Cerebral hemisphere (white matter)
    * In Children -> Brain stem
* Brain tumor having worst prognosis is glioblastoma multiformis.
* MC site of origin of oligodendroglioma is frontal lobe.
* Characteristic feature of oligodendroglioma are ,
    1. "Fried Egg" appearance
    2. PRone to **spontaneous hemorrhage.**

3. Calcification.

4. Dissemination through CSF.

* MC site of **choroid plexus papilloma** is :
    * In adult ->fourth ventricle
    * In children ->lateral ventricle
* MC site of CNS **lipoma** is corpus-callosum.
* MC site of intraspinal lipoma is thoracic region.
* MC abnormally associated with spinal lioma is **Spina Bifida.**
* MC type of Primitive Neuroectodermal tumors (PNET) is medulloblastoma.
* MC site of medulloblastoma is :
    * In adult -> Cerebellar hemisphere
    * In children -> Vermis of cerebellum.
* MC site for recurrence of medulloblastoma is posterior fossa.
* MC site of cranial ependymoma is fourth ventricle
* Mc site of spinal ependymoma is lumbar spine (Conus region).
* MC CNS tumor which occurs more frequently in women with breast cancer is meningioma.
* MC location of CNS meningioma is parasaggital
* Mc feature of parasaggital meningioma is spastic paraparesis and incontinence.
* Meningioma sometimes grow rapidly during pregnancy.
* Rosenthal fibres and microcysts are characteristics of pilocytic astrocytomas.
* Primary brain tumors, do not metastasise outside the CNS except,
    1. Glioblastoma
    2. Meduloblastoma.
* MC virus associated with primary CNS lymphoma in immunnocompromised patient is Epstein-barr virus.
* MC CNS tumor which causes polycythemia is hemangioblastoma.
* MC CNS tumor which gives rise to Diencephalic syndrome is Germinoma of Hypothalmic region.
* MC CNS tumor associated with Perinaud's syndrome is germinoma of pineal region.
* MC site of spinal meningioma is thoracic spine.
* MC cystic tumor, containing fluid resembling "Machinery oil" is craniopharyngiomas.

* MC site of CNS germinoma is pineal region
* MC tumor causing Foster-Kennedy syndrome is olfactory groove meningioma.
* Epidermoid tumors are also known as "Pearly tumors".
* MC site of chordoma is clivus.
* MC tumor of spinal cord is Schwannoma (Neurilemmoma).
* MC site of spinal neoplasm is thoracic cord.
* Most of spinal neoplasm are intradural extramedullary.
* MC site of spinal dermoid is **Lumbosacral area.**
* MC site for Neurofibroma is C1-2 interlaminar space.
* Most of spinal metastasis is extradural.
* MC cerebellopontine angle tumor is acoustic neuroma (second MC tumor is meningioma).
* MC nerve involved in Acoustic neurma is superior vestibular (8th Cr. Nerve)
* MC posterior fossa tumor of childhood having best prognosis is cerebellar astrocytoma.
* MC cranial nerve symptom in Brain stem glioma is diplopia & facial weakess.
* MC site of pilocytic astrocytoma is cerebellum.
* MC tumor of Peripheral nerve is Schwannoma (also called as perineurial fibroblastoma or neurilemmoma).
* MC presentation of peripheral nerve schwannoma is painless mass.
* MC symptoms of Brain tumor is **headache.**
* Sensory march of tonic-clonic seizure points to tumor of sensory parietal cortex.
* Brain tumors which contain FAT are
* MC agent which is used with MRI for contrast enhancement is godolinium DTPA.
* Contrast MRI provides definition of an altered blood-brain barrier.
* Echoplaner MRI (**Fast MRI**) provides assessment of blood volume within tumors.
* Investigation of choice for calcium containing meningiomas, Oligodendrogliomas and tumors of pineal region is **CT-SCAN.**
* TOC of the metastasis to skull base is **Radiotherapy.**

* TOC of Germinoma is **Radiotherapy.**
* Tumors which spread through CSF are,
  * Medulloblastoma
  * Oligodendroglioma
  * Germinoma
  * Glioblastoma (occaasionally)
  * Neuroblastoma.
* MC cause of solitary metastasis in brain is renal cell carcinoma.
* Tumors causing meningeal carcinomatosis includes,
  * Small cell CA of lung
  * Adenocarcinoma of lung.
  * CA. Breast
  * NHL (non-hodgkins lymphoma)
  * Leukemia
  * Melanoma.
* Drugs used to treat meningeal carcinomatosis are,
  * Thio-TEPA
  * Cytosine-arabinoside
  * Methotrexate
  * Methyl-prednisolone
* Cancers which spread to brain via paraspinal direct infiltration are,
  * Lymphoma
  * CA. prostate
  * CA-breast

ORBIT

* **MC** primary benign tumor of orbit is :
  * In infant and children   ->   CApillary Hemangioma
  * In adult   ->   Cavernous Hemangioma.
* Chocolate cysts of orbit is encysted blood in Lymphangiomas.
* MC primary malignant tumor of orbit in childhood is Rhabdomyosarcoma
  * MC primary tumors which gives rise to orbitl metastases,
  * In infant ->**Neuroblastoma** (usually bilaterla involvement of orbit)
  * In Children->Leukemia.
  * In adult ->
  1. Bronchogenic carcinoma (Male)
  2. Breast carcinoma (Female)

3. Hypermephroma
4. Prostatic carcinoma

* MC benign tumor of lacrymal gland is mixed cell tumor
* MC malignant tumor of lacrymal gland is adenoid cystic carcinoma (cylindroma)
* MC adjacent tumor which invades the orbit is sq. cell carcinoma of maxillary antrum.
* Demonstration of cross striations in the tumor cells is **pathognomic** of Rhabdomyosarcoma
* Racquet cells" or "Strap cells" are characteristic of **embryonal** form of Rhabdomyosarcoma.
* Most malignant type of Rhabdomyosarcoma is alveolar type
* MC type of Rhabdomyosarcoma is embryonal type
* Rarest type and having best prognosis of Rhabdomyosarcoma is pleomorphic type.
* Mc tumor of Lacrimal sac is Transitional cell tumor
* Tumor which is expansile & reducible and forms a gap in the underlying bone of orbit is meningo-encephalocele.
* MC part of orbit involved by Rhabdomyosarcoma is superonasal quadrant.

Conjunctiva and cornea

* MC tumor of conjunctiva is naevus (Benign pigment tumor).
* MC epibulbar tumor in children is choriostoma.
* MC site of conjunctival dermoid is **inferotemporal part** of the limbus.
* MC site of conjunctival naevus is limbus.
* MC site of epibulbar osseous choriostoma is **Superotemporal part** of bulbar conjunctiva.
* Complex choriostoma has a peculiar association with the linear sebaceous nevus of jadassohn.
* Mc site of squamous papilloma of conjunctiva in children is inferior fornix.
* Small sssile sq. papilloma of onjunctiva can be treated with **topical corticosteroid.**
* MC melanocytic tumor of conjunctiva is circumscribed nevus.
* MC site of the circumscribed nevus is **Interpalpebral bulbar conjunctiva.**
* MC site of malignant melanoma of conjunctiva is limbus.

* MC site of local metastasis from conjunctival malignant melanoma is regional lymph nodes.
* MC site of **distant** metastasis from conjunctival malignant melanoma is brain.
* Pyogenic granuloma of he conjunctiva is **neiher pyogenic nor** granulomatous but a proliferative fibrovascular response to prior tissue insult by inflammation, surgery or non-surgical trauma.
* Chocolate cysts" of conjunctiva is conjunctival lymph angioma.
* MC primary tumor which gives rise to secondary in conjunctiva is
  * Breast carcinoma in Female
  * Cutaneous melanoma in Male
* MC adjacent tumor from which conjunctiva is secondarily involved is sebaceous gland carcinomaof the eyelid.
* MC caruncular tumors are **papilloma & nevus.**
* MC site of benign Oncocytoma in eye is lacrymal glands.

Eyelids
* MC benign tumor of eyelid is squamous papilloma.
* Mc malignant tumor of eyelid is basal cell carcinoma.
* MC site of BCC is lower lid.
* MC site of SCC is lower lid margin.
* MC mesenchymal tumor of eyelid is hemangioma.
* Naevus flammeus is a capillary hemangioma.
* MC type of Basal cell carcinoma of lid is noduloulcerative type
* MC precancerous lesion of lid is actinic keratosis.
* MC type of Naevus in eyelid is intradermal naevus.
* MC site of sebaceous gland carcinoma (Meibomian cell carcinoma) is upper lid.
* Mc vascular tumor of eyelid is capillary hemangioma.
* Mc site for plexiform neurofibroma of eyelids are upper lid.

Malignant melanoma of choroid
* MC rimary intraocular tumor i.e. malignant melonoma of choroid
* Main primary intraocular disease that can be **fatal** in adults
* Median age of diagnosis is **55 yrs.**
* More common in **Males.**
* MC type of growth pattern is focal growth pattern
* Mc site of distant metastesis is liver.

RETINOBLASTOMA

* MC paediatric intraocular malignancy.
* Average age of diagnosis of retinoblastoma is 18 months (**rare after 7 yrs. of age).**
* Specific histologic finding of retinoblastoma.
  1. Flexiner-wintersteiner rossette.
  2. Fleuretes
* MC presenting pattern of growth in retinoblastoma is endophytic.
* MC clinial form of retinoblastoma is sporadic unilateral
* MC genetic form of retinoblastoma is somatic nonhereditory.
* MC endogenous mutagen in retinoblastoma is 5-methylcytosine
* Most widely used staging system of retinoblastoma is reeseellisworth classification.
* Most helpful and sensitive diagnostic test for retinoblastoma is **CT-SCAN** (Next best method is ultrasonography).
* MC cause of glaucoma in patient with rtinoblastoma is irisneovascularization.
* MC cause of pseudoretinoblastoma is persistent hyperplastic primary vitreous.
* The mainstay of conservative therapy of retinoblastoma is extrnal beam radiotherapy.
* Most radioresistant structure in the eye is sclera
* TOC in retinoblastoma, when tumor fills most of the globe and having very little or no hop of vision is enucleation.
* Most important factor to consider in enccleation in case of retinoblastoma is to **obtain a long stump of optic nerve.**
* **Cryotherapy** is useful for small tumor anterior to the equator when the tumor is mostly confined to the sensory retina.
* **Contraindications of cryotherapy :**
  1. Significant vitreous seeding.
  2. Tumors greater than 5 mm. in diameter and greater than 2.5 mm in thickness
* TOC of small retinoblastoma in the posterior pose is exenonarc photocoagulation.
* MC antineoplastic drug used in retinoblastoma is cyclophosphamide.
* **Trilateral retinoblastoma** consists of bilateral retinoblastoma with mid-line intracranial tumor (most commonly pineal gland tumors).
* MC hereditory cause of pseudoretinoblastoma is noorie's disease.

* Retinoma or retinocytoma is a benign varient of retinoblastoma.
* MC secondary tumor which develops in survivor of retinoblastoma is osteosarcoma.
* Calcification is an important **diagnostic** feature of the endophytic retinoblastoma.

                                                      Skull bone

* MC site of metastasis in retinoblastoma is ->Bone ——————
                                                    most commonly)

* A higher prevalence of retinoblastoma is reported with,
  * Trisomy-21
  * Deletion of long arm of the **D-chromosome.**

Miscellaneous points

* MC intraocualr malignancy is metastatic (secondaries).
* MC organ involved in secondaries to eye is CHOROID.
* MC primary which gives rise to secondary in eye is.
  * In Male   Lung cancer
  * In Female   Breast cancer
* Cluster of grapes" appearance is characteristic of cavernous hemangioma of the retina.
* Mc manifestation of Von-Hippel-Lindau syndrome is retinal capillary hemangioma.
* MD disease associated with retinal & optic nerve astrocytoma is tuberous sclerosis (Bourneville's disease, (JUXTA PULPILLRY REGION. .
* **MC site for Basal Cell Carcinoma of conjunctiva is PLICA-SEMILUNARIS**

THORAX

Benign Tumors

* MC bening tumor of chest wall is lipoma
* Mc benign neurogenic tumor of chest wall is solitary neurofibroma.
* MC benign skeletal tumor of chest wall is osteoma.
* MC site of **solitary fibrous dysplasia** is RIB.

Malignant Tumors

* MC primary soft tissue cancer of chest wall is fibrosarcoma.
* MC site of chondrosarcoma of chst wall is costochondral junction.
* Mc presentation of chondrosarcoma of chest wall is a **mass** (Not plain)

* Osteosarcoma of chest wall is **more malignant** than the chondrosarcoma
* Metastasis to the chest wall is often multiple and sites of primary tumor may be.
  * Thyroid
  * Breast
  * Kidney
  * Lung

TRACHEA

* MC tumor of trachea is the **direct extension** from a branchial, laryngeal, esophageal or thyroid primary.
* MC primary tumor of trachea is Sq. cell carcinoma and adenoid cystic carcinoma.
* MC **benign** tumor of trachea in **children** is hemangioma
* TOC of tracheal neoplasm is endoscopic laser ablation.
* Most useful laser utilised for endoscopic ablation of tracheal neoplasm is **Nd-YAG-LASER.**
* **Photodynamic therapy** using Argon laser beam is also used for treatment.
* Tumoricidal agent **used in** Photodynamic therapy is **Hematoporphyrin** derivatives.
* To minimise the tension on the anastomosis in case of trachea reconstruction operation the neck is hold in **hyperextension** for at least 7 days postoperatively.

Mediastinum

* MC mediastinal malignancy is **lymphoma** .
* MC mass lesions of **Anterior** mediastinum in **adult is thymoma** (if general, it is lymphoma).
* MC mass lesions of **middle** mediatinum is vascular masses.
* MC mass lesions of **Posterior** mediastinum is neurogenic tummors.
* M/C mediastinal neutrogenic tumor is Schwannoma (Neurilemoma).
* MC type of thymoma is epithelial type
* MC type of thymoma associated with myasthenia gravis is lymphocytic tyre.
* MC approach for thymomectomy is though **median sternotomy.**
* MC approach for remova of neurogenic tumor is posterolateral thoracotomy

* TOC of lymphoma is radiation
* MC site of extragonodal teratoma **in adult is anterior medias-tinum**
* MC structure involved in adhesion from a teratodermoid tumor in the mediastinum is pericardium
* Mc mesenchymal tumor of mediastinum is lipoma
* MC site for mediastinal mesenchymal tumor is anterio mediastinum.
* MC site for mediastinal mesenchymal tumor is anterior mediastinum
* MC lymph-vascular tumr of mesiadtinum is lymphangioma (cystic hygroma).
* MC primary mediastinal cyst is -Pericardial (Ref. SChwartz-p. 768
* MC site of Bronchogenic cyst is **just posterior to the carina.**
* MC site of **Enteric cyst** of mediastinum is posterior mediastinum
* MC thymic abnormality associated with myesthenia gravis is formation of germinal center (Next abnormality->Thymoma
* Thymomectomy is now recommended for all patients with myesthenia gravis whether or not a thymoma is present.
* Most valuable imaging teachnique for mediastinum is CT-scan
* **Definitive diagnosis** is done by Mediastinoscopy.
* MC site of primary which gives rise to metastatis in the mediastinum is
  1. From **adjacent** source-> Bronchogenic carcinoma
2. From distant source -CA breast, tumor is cells of kulchitsky located in the Thymus.
* MC site of **Giant Lymph Node Hyperplasia** (Castleman's Disease), is mediastinum.
* MC mediastinal cysts associated wtih congenital abnormaliteis of the vertebrae are Enterogenous (ENTERIC) cyst.
* Pericadial cystic are also called as :
  * **Spinrogwater cysts**
  * **Mesotheula cysts.**
* MC tumor of pleura is **Metastatic carcinoma** (secondaries).
* MC source of secondaries on pleura are cancers of Lung & Breast.
* MC primary tumor of pleura is **mesothelioma.**
* MC primary benign tumor of plrua is **Spindle cell tyre of** localised mesothelioma.
* MC primary malignant tumor of pleura is diffuse -epithelial malignant mesothelioma.
* MC situ of mesothelioma in the body is pleura (other is Peritoneum & Pericardium).

* MC predisposing factors for plerual mesothelioma is exposure to **Asbestos.**
* Mc variety of astbestos responsible for mesothelioma is AMP-Hibole (not serpentine).
* Mc Histological type of Mesothelioma is Biphasic type (having both sarcomatoid and epitheloid areas).
* MC site involved in distant spread from malignant mesothelioma is liver.
* TOC of benign (localised) mesothelioma is local excision.
* MC type of **monoclonal antibody** used for diagnosis of accurate histology of malignant mesothelioma is **ME-1.**
* Benign mesothelioma may be associated with hypoglycemia.
* Malignant mesothelioma may be associated with thrombocytosis which accounts for high incidence of thromboembolic phenomenon.
* Drugs used for **Pleurodesis** (adhesion between parietal & visceral pleura0 are :
  * Quinacrine
  * Minocyclin (tetracyclin)
  * Bleomycin
  * Talc
* MC antineoplastic drug used for maligant mesothelioma is doxorubicin **(Adriamycin).**

Heart, pericardium & Diaphragm

* MC cardiac tumors are secondaries (Metastatic tumor).
* MC primary neoplasm of heart is Myxoma.
* Mc primary benign tumor in adult is myxoma
* MC primary benign cardiac tumor in infant & children is rhabdomyoma.
* MC site of myxoma in heart is left atrium.
* Mc malignant tumor of heart is sarcoma (usually angiosarcoma and Rhabdomyosarcoma)
* MC site of malignant sarcoma is right atrium.
* "Spider cells" are seen in Rhabdomyoma.
* Tumor plop and Positional alterations of murmur is considered diagnostic of myxoma.
* MC primaries which give rise to metastases in heart include,
  * Lung carcinoma (commonest in male)
  * Breast carcinoma (commonest in female)
  * Malignant melanoma
  * Lymphoma
  * Leukemia.

* All areas of heart can be involved in metastatic deposit except cardiac valves (due to absence of lymphatics in valves)
* MC primary benign tumor of pericardium is teratoma.
* MC primary malignant tumor of pericardium is mesothelioma.
* MC tumor of pericardium is metastatic (secondaries).
* MC tumor of diaphragm is metastatic (secondaries).
* MC primary benign tumor of diaphragm is lipoma.
* MC primary malignant tumor of diaphragm is fibrosarcoma.

Lung

* MC tumor of lung is primary malignant tumor (carcinoma).
* Mc benign tumor of lung is hamartoma (chondroadenoma).
* "Popcorn calcification" is **pathognomonic** findings of pulmonary harmartomas.
* Clubbing or Hypertrophic osteoarthropathy does not occur in benign tumor of the lung except in fibrous-mesotheliomas.
* Marable like feel of the tumor is **characteristic** of pulmonary hamartoma.
* MC cause of **recurrent hemoptysis** is bronchial adenoma.

Carcinoma Lung

* MC cause of cancer death in **both** men & women.
* MC cancer of lung in wild is adenocarcinoma.
* MC cancer of lung **in India is** Sq. cell carcinoma.
* MC risk factor responsible for lung cancer is smoking
* MC lung cancer found in nonsmoker is adenocarcinoma.
* MC environmental pollutants of natural origina responsible for lung cancer is Radon Gas.
* MC associated paraneoplastic syndrome with sq. cell Ca lung is hypercalcemia and Hypophosphatemia
* Have **highest resectibility** rate.
* MC molecular genetic abnormality is **over expression of epidermal growth factor receptor (EGFR).**
* MC molecular genetic abnormality is over expression of epidermal growth factor receptor (EGFR)
* **Bronchoalveolar** (type)
* MC cancer arises from a pulmonary scar (especially, Bronchoalveolar type).
* MC cancr that may be spread by Aerosol Transmission (especially , Bronchoalveolar type.

* MC associated skeletal connective tissue syndrome is Hypertrophic pulmonary osteoarthropathy.
* MC molecular genetic abnormally to mutation of K-rass oncogene.
* MC molecular genetic abnormalities are,
  * Amplicication of the myc-oncogene family
  * Mutation of rat-gene
  * Deletion of short arm of chromosome 3 (3p)
* MC type of lung cancer associatd with paraneoplastic and skeletal connective tissue syndrome.
* MC lung carcinoma having **extrathoracic metastases.**
* **The main patholgoy in Eaton-Lambert syndrome is development of antivoltage gated calcium channel antibodies.**
* **MC nerves involved in Pancoast syndrome if** C8T1,2-
* MC structures destroyed in Pancoast syndrome is **First and second ribs.**
* MC symptom of lung cancer is cough.
* MC site of distant metastasis is liver.
* Investigation of choice for mediastinal involvement.
* **Contraindications of Radiation Therapy in Ca lung are :**
  8 Extrathoracic distant metastases.
  * Positive supraclavicula nodes
  * Malignant pleural effusion.
  * Cardiac involvement

BREAST

CARCINOMA OF THE FEMALE BREAST
* MC cause of cancer of female in **developed countries.**
  (in India it is CA. cervix)
* Second MC cause of cancer death in female (after CA. Lung).
* MC type of breast carcinoma is scirrhous type of infltrating (invasive) ductal adenocarcinoma.
* Also known as not otherwise specific type
* MC site of carcinoma in breast is upper outer quadrant.
* Mc site of distant metastasis is bone
* MC sign & symptom of breast carcinoma is palpable mass.

Risk Factors
* Old age

* White race.
* Unmarried.
* Nulliparity & infertility.
* Early menarche (< 12 yrs).
* Late menopuse (>50 yrs.)
* Obesity
* History of cancer is one breast.
* History of benign prolifrative lesins.
* Any first degree relative with history of breast cancer.
* Mother & sister with history of breast cancer.
* History of Primary cancer in endometrium or ovary
* Large dose of radiation therapy to chest.
* Dysplastic mammographic parenchymal pattern (**Mammary dysplasia).**
* Increased fat content in diet.
* Very high dose of estrogen therapy in postmenopausal women.
* High socioeconomic status
* Moderate alcohol intake.
* **Most curable** of all breast cancers are those associated with such microcalcification patter on mammography.
* **The sensitivity** of mammography is approx. **60-90%**
* The specificity of mammography is :
  (i) · for nonpalpable mammographic abnormalities -> 30-40% (approx)
  (ii) for clinically evident malignancies - 85-90% (Approx).
* **Failure** of mammography is seen in cases of :
  (i) Clinical cancer in a very **dense breast.**
  (ii) **Young women** with mammary dysplasia.
  (iii) **Medullary** type of breast carcinoma
* Mammography is never a substitute for biopsy, so biopsy must be followed after mammography.
* MC type of mammography utilized in breast cancer is Film screen mammography (not xeromammography) because of less delivery of radiation.
* Cardiomyopathy due to toxicity of Doxorubcin occurs when the comulative dose exceed 450 mg/m2 body area.
* Patient with a larger breast mas or a higher clinical stage are more likely to have positive nodes.
* In general breast cancer appears to be somewhat more malignant in younger than in olde women

* Indian file patern and bulls eye pattern of cellular arrangement is characteristic.
* Brest is diffusely "Brawny" and nipple is often retracted.

Carcinoma of male breast

* MC type is infiltrating ductal carcinoma.
* **Predisposing risk factors :**
    * Klinefelter syndrome
    * Testicular feminizing syndrome
* Estrogen therapy
    * Radiation exposure
    * A family history of brest cancer
    * Schistosomiasis
    * Trauma
* Nipple discharge is an omnious finding in Ca breast in male.
* MC site for distant metastases is bone
* Hormone dependence is typical and tumor is commonly ER-positive
* MC site of primary cancer which gives rise to secondary in male breast is prostate

Other Breast tumors

* MC benign tumor of breast is fibroadenoma
* MC tumor of breast below the age 30 years if fibroadenoma
* TOC of fibroadenoma is excisional biopsy
* Cystosarcoma phylloid is a **giant intracanalicular fibroadenoma**
* 'Teardrop' configuration is seen in cystosarcoma phylloid.
* TOC of benign cystosarcoma phylloid is wide excision
* TOC of Malignant cystosarcoma phylloid is simple mastectomy.
* Second MC solid tumor of breast is fibroadenoam (First is CA-breast)
* "Cut cabbage" configuration is seen in **cystosarcoma phylloides.**
* MC site of metastasis in Angiosarcoma & Malignant cystosarcoma phylloides is **Lung.**
* MC cause of bloody nipple discharge is benign intraductal papilloma.
* MC cause of nipple discharge is benign duct ectasia.
* MC cause of breast tendernes of fibrocystic disease.
* Li-fraument syndrome : It comprises high risk of certain cancrs due to inherited mutation of tumor suppressor gene P53 in some families.
    * High risk cancers includes,
        1. Lung carcinoma
        2. Breast carcinoma

Papillary carcinoma

* MC type of thyroid carcinoma
* MC type of thyroid carcinoma developed in previously radiation exposed thyroid glands.
* Presence of "Orphan annie nuclei" in papillary Ca thyroid
* Presence of Psammoma bodies.
* Hurthle cells have eosinophilic cytoplasm heavily packed with mitochondria.
* MC site of distant metastases is lung
* Metastases in bone is frequently osteoblastic
* Mc tumor marker is calcitonin.
* MC symptom of medulary Ca thyroid is diarrhoea.
* Only thyroid cancer that is associated with cushing's syndrome.
* Patients with men syndrome have defect in **Chromosome -10.**
* MC presenting feature in thyroid cancer is goitre.
* MC sites of primary from where secondaries reach the thyroid gland are.
1. Kidney (Hypernephroma)
2. Lung (Bronchogenic carcinoma)

Other tumors of thyroid

* MC cause of solitary thyroid nodule is follicular adenoma.
* MC benign tumor of thyroid is adenoma.
* MC type of thyroid adenoma is follicular adenoma.
* MC type of solitary thyroid nodule is colloid nodule (Ref. Schwartz. P.1632).
* A thyroid mass must reach the size of 1 cm to become palpable clinically.
* Malignant lymphoma of thyroid sometime develops in Autoimmune thyroiditis (Hashimoto's thyroiditis).
* Type of malignant lymphoma arises in thyroid gland is usually Non-Hodgkins Lymphoma

Pituitary Gland

* MC tumor of pituitary is adenoma
* Microadenoma is adenoma < 10 mm in diameter
* Macroadenomais adenoma > 10 mm in diameter.
* MC functional pituitary tumors are prolactinomas.
* MC symptoms of prolactinoma in female is secondary amenorrhea
* MC symptom of prolactinoma in male is decreased libido.
* Second MC pituitary adenoma is null cell adenoma.

* MC pituitary adenoma is sparsely granulated prolactinoma.
* Largest pituitary adenoma is somatotroph (GH Cell) adenoma.
* MC nonfunctioning pituitary adenoma is nononcocytic, Null-cell adenoma.
* MC cause of non-physiologic hypersecretion of prolactin is prolactinoma.
* MC pituitary adenoma responsible for amenorrheagalactorrhea syndrome is prolactinoma.
* MC cause of hyperpituitarism is adenoma
* MC cause of bitemporal hemianopia is chromophobe pituitary adenoma.
* 'Ape Man' of the circus is produced by acidophilic (eosiniphilic) pituitary adenoma.
* MC presentation of Adrenal cortical carcinoma is Cushing's syndrome.
* MC drug used for palliative treatment of Adrenal cortical carcinoma is Mototane. (Other drug is Doxorubicin)
* MC cause of feminization is adrenal cortical carcinoma
* Incidentalomas are non-functioning adenomas discovered incidentally after examination of abdomen for various diseases.
* MC site of primary cancer which gives rise to secondary in the adrenal gland is lung.
* MC cause of virilization is congenital adrenal hyperplasia
* MC cause of primary hyperaldosteronism is adrenal cortical adenoma.
* MC site for distant spread in Adrenal cortial carcinoma is Lung.

Pheochromocytoma
* MC site of origin is adrenal medulla.
* Paragangliomas are extra adrenal pheochromocytoma that originates from.
  * Giands of zuckerkandi (at the bifurcation of the aorta)->most common
  * Lumbar paravertebral ganglia
  * Preaortic ganglia
  * Thorocic paravertebral ganglia
  * Urinary bladder
  * Pelvis
  * Renal hilum
  * Skull
  * Chest or neck
  * Pericardium
  * Vagina
  * Mediastinum

* MC manifestation (Sign) of pheochromocytoma is hypertension.
* MC is young to mid-adult life.
* Mc symptoms of pheochromocytoma is headache.
* MC neuroectodermal disease associated with pheochromocytoma is neurofibromatosis.
* Zellballen" : is histologically the ball like aggregates, representing the tumor cells disposed in nests or cords separated by a vasculrized connective tissue stroma.
* Best screening test for pheochromocytoma is the measurement of 24 hour urinary metanephrine.
* **Drug of choice** to reduce hypertension during operation is sodium nitriprusside or phenotolamine.
* β-blockers are used to treat a patient with pheochromocytoma only
* β-blockers should never be administered without prior alpha-adrenergic blockage in pheochromocytoma.
* MC approach for surgery in pheochromocytoma is anterior transabdominal approach
* MC structure which must be ligated early in the operation to avoid a sudden influx of catecholamine during tumor removal is adrenal vein.
* MC metabolic abnormality which may develop after operation in a patient of pheochromocytoma is hypoglycemia.
* MC site of metastases of malignant pheochromocytoma should be followed yearly.
* MC site of metastases of malignant pheochromocytoma is bone & lung.
* Treatment of pheochromocytoma in Early pregnancy is the surgical removal as soon as the diagnosis is confirmed, provided that the patient is prepared with phenoxy benzamine preoperatively.
* Malignant pheochromocytomas are more common in children and in extra-adrenal tumors.
* First biochemical abnormality detected in MEN-I is hyperparathyroidism.
* MC manifestation is hypercalcemia.
* Second MC expression of MEN-I is neoplasia of the Pancreatic islet cells (MC is parathyroid hyperplasia).
* MC pancreatic islet-cell lesion in patient with MEN-I is PPOMA (secretion of **Pancreatic polypeptide).**
* Second MC pancreatic islet cell neoplasm in patient with MEN-I is gastrinoma.
* MC cause of death in patient having MEN-I is pancreatic involvement.

* MC pathology of pancreas in MEN I is carcinoma.
* MC pathology of pituitary involvement is Prolactin-secreting microadenoma.
* MC pathology in MEN IIA is Medullary Ca of thyroid.
* First abnormality detected is Medullary CA of thyroid.
* MC pathology in parathyroid involvement is chief cell hyperplasia.
* The pheochromocytomas are nearly always limitd to the adrenal medulla, nearly always benign and nearly **always bilateral.**
* Non endocrine manifestatins of MEN II B:
  1. "Marfanoid body habitus"
  2. Mucosal neuroma ('Bumpy lips')
  3. Multiple mucocutaneous ganglioneuromas of GIT.

GIT

Benign Tumors
* MC benign esophageal tumor is leiomyoblastoma (Leiomoma).
* MC site of leiomyomas are lwoer 2/3rd of esophagus.
* Leiomyomas are more common males.
* MC symptoms of leiomyomas are dysphagia and pain.
* Most useful method to demonstrate a leiomyoma of esophagus is barium swallow.
* TOC of leiomyoma -> simple enucleation.

CA Esophagus
* MC Malignant tumor of esophagus -> sq cell. carcinoma
* MC site of Ca esophagus = **Middle Third.**
* MC site of **adenocarcinoma** of esophagus -> Barret's esophagus.
* MC early symptoms of esophageal cancer -> **Progressive Dysphagia**
* MC early symptom of tumors cardia -**Anorexia and wt. loss.**
* MC site of metastasis is adjacent and supracalvicular lymph nodes.
* MC anticancer drugs use as single drug rgimen in Tt. of CA. esophagus is cisplatin.
* MC other drug used with cisplatin as combined chemotherapy in Tt. of CA esophagus = 5-Fluorouracil
* MC cause of failure in patient treated with preoperative chemotherapy is the emergence of systemic disease.

STOMACH

Benign Tumors

* MC benign tumor of stomach is Polyp (Papillary excrescences of gastric epithelium)
* MC malignant tumor of stomach is **adenocarcinoma.**
* MC sign of gatric cancer is anorexia with weight loss.
* MC symptom of gastric cancer is upper abdominal discomfort.
* MC clinical type of Ca stomach is Advanced Carcinoma (25%)
* MC site of gastric cancer-Pre-pyloric region
* MC site for hematogenous spread of tumor = Liver.
* Most important dietary factor responsible for gastric carcinoma is **Nitrate** in dried, smoked and salted food.
* Nitrate is converted in carcinogenic **nitrites** by endogenous bacteria such as **H. Pylori** or Exogenous bacteria through contaminated food.
* Most frequent extranodal location of lymphoma is **stomach**
* MC type of gastric lymphoma ->**Non-Hodkin's lymphoma of B-cell origin.**
* MC presenting complaint of gastric lymphoma is **anorexia and** wt. loss.
* MC gastric sarcoma -> **Leiomyosarcoma.**
* MC site of leiomyosarcoma->**Anterior & posterior** walls of the gastric **fundus.**
* **Leiomyosarcoma** donot **metastasize to lymph nodes.**
* MC site of metastases in leiomyosarcoma is **Liver & Lung.**
* TOC of leiomyosarcoma->**Surgical resection.**
* MC benign tumor of small intestine->**Adenoma.**
* MC benign tumor of small intestine that produces symptoms -leiomyoma.
* MC site of adenoma in small intestine is ileum.
* MC site of villous adenoma in GIT is duodenum.
* MC site of Brunner's gland adenoma is **duodenum.**
* MC site of leiomyoma is **jejunum.**
* MC site of Lipoma is **ileum** (distal part) & Ileocecal valve.
* MC site of isolated hemangioma is **jejunum.**
* MC clinical manifestations of small bowel tumors are **Bleeding & Obstruction.**
* MC benign tumors causing bleeding is **Leiomyomas & Hemangiomas.**
* MC treatment applied for benign small bowel tumor is **segmental resection** and **primary reanastomosis.**

* MC complications of benign neoplasm requiring treatments are Bleeding & Obstruction.
* MC indication for operation on leiomyoma is **Bleeding.**
* MC benign neoplasm of small intestine found at the leading point of an intussuception is Lipoma.
* MC primary cancer of small bowel is adenocarcinoma (50%)
* MC site of small bowel cancer is Distal Duodenum & Proximal Jejunum
* MC presenting symptom of periampullary adenocarcinoma is **Intermittent Jaundice.**
* Mc sarcoma of small intestine is **Leiomyosarcoma.**
* MC indications for operation in case of leiomyosarcoma of small intestine is bleeding & obstruction.
* MC site of small bowel lymphoma is Ileum.
* MC site of primary lymphoma from which secondary small intestinal lymphoma develops - **Retroperitoneal Lymph Nodes.**
* Most prominent humoral agents secreted by carcinoid tumors are **serotonin & substance-P.**
* MC symptoms are **abd. pain.** bowel obstruction, diarrhoea and weight loss.
* Angiography is the **most sensitive** diagnostic test to detect hepatic metastasis.
* Most effective method for preventing colon cancer is to remove the colon once dysplasia has been identified.
* Most accurate method to detect metastasis in liver is **Angio-CT Scanning** (Sensitivity is 95% approx.).

Carcinoma Colon

* MC symptoms of CA of **right** colon is related to symptoms of **anemia** due to chronic blood loss.
* MC symptoms of CA **left** colon - change in bowel habit.
* MC site is rectosigmoid junction.
* CA colon is more common on left-side.
* Left sided tumors of colon are **obstructive** (Annular type).

Carcinoma Rectum

* MC type is adenocarcinoma
* MC and earliest symptoms -Bleeding per rectum.
* Mc specific symptoms of Ca rectum early morning diarrhoea.
* The most unique aspect of anatomy of the rectum is its easy accessibility.
* Extent of fixation of the tumor is an important predictor of prognosis.

* Signet ring cells & mucinous cancers are very aggressive histologic pattern of rectal cancers.

Miscellaneous points about colorectal tumors

* MC sites of colorectal involvement of lymphomas are caecum & rectum.
* Fish flesh appearance of cut surface is found in case of GIT lymphoma.
* TOC of Colorectal lymphoma-complete excision.
* Colonic lymphoma is more common in male.
* Rectal lymphoma is more common in female.
* MC type of colonic lymphoma is histiocytic NHL.
* Colonic carcinoids of <1 cm are usually asymptomatic and never malignant.
* Overall 5-year survival rate for colonic **carcinoid is less than 50%**
* **Alpha-interferon** is used in Tt. of malignnat carcinoid of colon.
* MC site of composite carcinoid-carcinoma (adenocarcinoid) is appendix.
* MC malignant tumors found in retrorectal space is chordomas.
* Bony destruction in chordomas usually indicate malignancy.
* Treatment of choice of chordoma is **surgical resection.**
* **Scimitar's Sign** (sacrum with rounded, concave border without bony destruction) is the pathognomonic X-ray appearance of anterior sacral meningoceles.
* MC site of distant metastasis is liver.
* Carcinoma distal to pectinate line ulcerates more frequently.
* Anal canal is the third most common site for melanoma (following skin and eye).
* MC D/D of melanoma of anal canal is thrombosed piles.
* MC site of lymph node metastasis in melanoma of anal canal ismesenteric lymph nodes.
* MC site of visceral metastasis of anal canal melanoma is lung.
  Melanoma of anal canal is **radioresistant,** so surgery is the treatment of choice.

Liver

* Malignant changes do not occur in hemangioma.
* In adult, most hepatic hemangiomas should not be excised.
* Angiogram demonstrate typical sunburst, hypervasculr pattern in focal nodular hyperplasia of in nodular hyperplasia of liver
* A radionucleotide technetium scan usually show a hot spot because of the presence of Kupffer cells.

* Type of cirrhosis having highest risk of developing hepatocellular carcinoma is post-necrotic cirrhosis (associated with HBV infection)
* Type of cirrhosis having lowest risk is alcoholic cirrhosis.
* MC presenting symptoms of hepatocellular Ca liver are abdominal pain & weight loss.

Types of metastasis :
* Precocious metastasis :
    * When the primary lesion is not suspected.
    * Example :-Carcinoid tumor of ileum.
* Synchronous metastasis :
    * When the hepatic neoplasm is detected at the same time as the primary lesion
* Metachronous metastasis :
    * Appearance is delayed following the successful removal of a parimary tumor.
    * Example : - Ocular melanoma.
* MC lab. finding is increased serum alkaline phosphatse level.

Carcinoma of Gall Ballader
* MC malignant lesion of the biliary tract
* MC type of Ca GB is scirrhous adenocarcinoma.
* 90% cases are associated wtih gall stones.
* MC symptom in Ca GB is unremitting right upper quadrant pain.
* MC operation performed in circinoma gall bladder is exploration & biopsy as most patients will have incurable & unresectable disease at the time of presentation.
* MC site of venous metastasis is quadrate lbe of liver (segment IV)
* Highest degree of diagnostic accuracy in Ca GB is provided by Angiography.
* MC presenting feature of Ca extrahepatic bile duct is jaundice (obstructive.
* MC means of diagnosis is cholangiography following ultrasound demonstration of dilated intrahepatic bile duct.
* Klatskin tumor : It is a nodular form of cholangio-carcinoma which arises at the confluence of right & left hepatic duct.

Cancer of exocrine pancreas
* MC type of Ca exocrine pancreas is ductal adenocarcinoma
* MC site is head of the pancreas.
* MC presenting feature is abdominal pain.

* MC cause of wt. loss is anorexia (not malabsorption).
* Most consistently observed risk factor for Ca pancreas is smoking.
* Characteristic finding suggesting diagnosis of Ca pancreas is a constriction of, both the pancreatic bile ducts in the head of the gland. So this is called double-duct sign.
* Whipple's triad is classical diagnostic criteria which consists of
  1. Hypoglycemic symptoms produced by fasting.
  2. Blood glucose concentration below 50mg/dL during symptomatic episodes, and
  3. Relief of symptom following intravenous administration of glucose.

Gastrinoma
* (Zollinger-Ellison syndrome)
* MC site of gastrinoma is pancreas (80%) mc site in pancreas is the head.
* Most commonly arises from Non-beta cells of pancreatic islets.
* MC site of Vipoma is body or Tail of Pancreas.

Somatostatinoma
* Arises from delta cells of pancreatic islets.
* Triad of somatostatinoma includes :
  1. Diabetes mellitus (mild).
  2. Steatorhoea, and
  3. Cholelithiasis.
* MC site of somatostatinoma is pancreas (2nd MC site is small intestine).

Glucagonoma
* Glucagonoma arises from alpha-cells (more precisely α_2 of pancreatic islets.
* Tumors are single, large, slow growing, more than 75% have metastasized at the time of diagnosis.
* MC sites of metastasis are liver & bones.
* The hallmarks of the glucagonoma syndrome are **mild diabetes & severe dermatitis.**
* MC site of skin lesion in glucagonoma is face.

Urogenital system
Kidney
* MC benign solid parenchymal tumor is adenoma.

* Spoke-wheel pattern on angiography is typical of Renal oncocytoma (due to central stellate scar).
* MC benign tumor in newborn and infant is mesoblastic nephroma (fetal hamartoma).
* Benign tumor associated with tuberous sclerosis is angiomyolipoma (hamartoma).
* MC site for renal hemangioma is renal pelvis

Malignant Tumors
* Primary, and
* Secondary

Primary Malignant Tumors of Renal Parenchyma :
1. Epithelial tissue origin :
   (i) Renal cell carcinoma
   (ii) Renal papillary carcinoma
2. Embryonal tissue origin :
   (i) Wilm's tumor or Embryonal adenomyosarcoma.
3. Connective tissue (interstitial tissue) origin :
   (i) Fibrosarcoma
   (ii) Liposarcoma
   (iii) Leiomyosarcoma.
* MC neoplasm of kidney
* MC site of origin of renal cell carcinoma is prox. convoluted tubule earliest and MC presenting feature is intermittent painless, gross or microscopic hematuria (total hematuria).
* MC site of distant metastasis is lung (cannon Ball secondaries, secondaries may be pulsatile).
* MC route of distant metastasis is hematogenous.
* Diagnostic procedure of choice in renal cell Ca is CT-scan.
* Most accurate noninvasive means of detecting renal vein or venacaval thrombi is MRI.
* Stauffer's syndrome is hepatic cell dysfunction in renal cell carcinoma.
* Classical triad of renal cell carcinoma consists of
  1. Gross hematuria
  2. Flank pain
  3. Palpable abdominal mass.
* Specific X-ray finding suggestive of malignant renal tumor mass is central calcification.

Renal Sarcoma

* MC sarcoma of kidney is leiomyosarcoma.
* MC sites of primary tumors giving rise to secondary renal deposits are :
  1. Lung
  2. Stomach
  3. Breast

RENAL PELVIS & CALICES

* MC tumor is urothelial transition cell carcinoma.
* Least common and having worst prognosis, tumor is sq. cell CA of renal pelvis.
* MC presenting feature is gross or microscopic painless hematuria.
* Sq. cell CA is most commonly associated with chronic inflammation and stone formation.
* Transitional cell CA is usually **avascular** on arteriography.

URETER

* MC tumor of ureter is transitional cell CA.
* MC site is lower ureter.
* MC presenting feature is gross or microscopic hematuria.
* Bladder cancer is the **second** most common cancer of the genitourinary tract and the most common cancer of urinary collecting system.
* MC cancer is transitional cell carcinoma.
* MC type of transitional cell carcinoma is superficial type.
* MC site is trigone and the adjacent posterolateral wall.
* MC presenting complaint is gross and microscopic hematuria.
* Sq. cell CA is the most common bladder cancer in chronic inflammation due to :
  * Schistomiasis, and
  * Calculus

Carcinoma Prostate

* MC cancer (excluding skin cancer) in adult male (In India, CA, Oral cavity is the MC cancer).
* Third MC cause of cancer death (after long and colon)
* MC malignancy in men over 55 yrs. of age is Ca prostate.
* MC type is adenocarcinoma.
* MC site is **Posterior lobe.**
* In symptomatic patient, MC presenting complaint in Ca prostate is dysuria.

* Most appropriate test for detection of all stages of Ca prostate (except stage A) is digital rectal examination.
* Most accurate diagnostic imaging study for CA prostate is transrectal ultrasound (trus).
* Most reliable procedure for pelvic staging in Ca prostate is pelvic lymphadenectomy by laparoscopic approach.
* Most sensitive test for early detection of CA prostate is elevated serum Prostate Specific Antigen (PSA) level.
* Confirmatory test to diagnose CA prostate is **Needle Biopsy.**
* MRI appears to be more helpful in pelvic stagin than CT-scan.
* Magnetic resonance spectroscopy shows differences in phosphocreatine/ATP and citrate/lactate ratios in benign vs. malignant prostate cancer.
* Cyt-356, a monoclonal antibody, coupled with a radio-isotope is used for diagnosis of soft tissue and bone **metastasis** in Ca prostate.
* PSA is most useful in following patients, after treatment.
* Mc site of lymphatic metastasis is obturator lymph node.
* MC site of hematogenous metastasis is pelvic bone.
* MC site of visceral metastasis is lung.
* Suramin, a growth factor inhibitor is investigational agent in the treatment of metastatic prostatic CA.

CA. URETHRA

* MC type is **sq. cell carcinoma**
* More common in females than males.
* MC site of male is bulbomembranous urethra.
* MC symptom in female in Ca urethra is urethral bleeding. MC symptom in male is abnormal urethral discharge.
* Treatment & Prognosis :
* MC testicualr tumor in children is **yolk sac** tumor.
* MC testicular tumors are **germinal cell** tumors.
* Germinal cell tumors are almost always **malignant.**
* Stromal cell tumors are usually benign.
* MC malignant germ cell tumor is seminoma.
* MC tumor arising from undescended testis is seminoma.

Carcinoma Penis

* MC site is glans penis or, foreskin (prepuce).
* MC type is squamous cell carcinoma.

* Adenocarcinoma of penis arises from **gland of Tyson.**
* MC site of metastasis is inguinal lymph nodes.
* MC presentation in Ca penis is an exophytic nodular or wartlike growth with secondary infection.
* Earliest symptoms are a mild irritation and a purulent discharge from the prepuce.

GYNAECOLOGY

Leiomyoma of Uterus

* MC benign solid tumor in female.
* MC benign tumor of uterus.
* MC location is body of the uterus.
* MC type is intramural
* Wandering fibroid (parasitic fibroid) is a type of subserous fibroid which get detached from the uterus and takes nourishment from the adjacent viscera (usually omentum).
* Degneration in myoma starts from the middle portion, while calcification begins from the periphery.
* MC secondary changes taking place in myoma is degeneration.
* MC type of degeneration is hyaline degeneration.
* MC site of degeneration is the centre.
* MC D/D of cystic degeneration of fibroid is lymphangiectasis.
* Calcareous degeneration is most common insubserous fibroid.
* Womb-stone is completely calcified, sessile, subserous myoma.
* MC condition associated with Red degeneration of fibroid is pregnancy.
* Red degeneration is also called as carneous degeneration.
* Red degeneratio is most common during second half (especially, third trimester) of pregnancy and puerpurium.
* 'Fishy odour' is characteristic of Red degeneration.
* MC type of myoma having higher potential for sarcomatous change is Intramural & Submucous.
* Most important sign of sarcomatous changes in myoma is non-encapsulaion of the tumor.
* Torsion is most commonly seen in subserous myoma.
* Inversion of uterus is MC in submucous myoma.
* Infection arises most frequently in submucous myomas & myomatous polypi.

* Infertility is most common in submucous myoma.
* MC symptom of myoma is menorrhagia.
* Metrorrhagia is MC in Submucous myoma.
* Pseudo-meigs syndrome is most commonly caused by subserous myoma.
* MC myoma which is easily removed by myomectomy is subserous type.
* Bonney's Hood operation is indicated for removal of Fundal fibroid.
* MC germ cell tumor of ovary is dermoid cyst (Benign cystic teratoma).
* Rokitansky's protruberence is seen in Dermoid cysts.
* MC ovarian tumor found during pregnancy is dermoid cysts.
* **Meigs' syndrome** is the association of Ascites and right sided hydrothorax with **benign** tumors of ovary.
* MC ovarian tumor associated with Meiges' syndrome is fibroma.
* MC ovarian malignant tumor associated wtih Pseudo-meigs' syndrome is Brenner's tumor & Granulosa cell tumor.
* MC benign ovarian tumor of connective tissue origin is fibroma.
* MC complication of benign cystic ovarian tumor is torsion of the pedicle.
* Malignancy is lowest in dermoid cyst and usually a squamous cell carcinoma.
* MC type of cyst lying anterior to uterus is Dermoid Cyst.
* MC complication of immature teratoma is malignant transformation.

Other Benign Tumors
* MC location of hidradenoma is **anterior part of labia majora.**
* TOC of hidradenoma is local excision.
* MC tumor of Broad ligment & parametrium is Myoma.
* MC site of Gartner's duct cyst is anterolateral wall of vagina.
* MC site of Epithelial inclusion cyst is lower 1/3rd of vagina on the posterior wall.
* MC site of vaginal endometriotic cyst is posterior vaginal wall behind the cervix (Posterior fornix).
* MC type of benign uterine polyp is Mucous polyp.
* Malignancy arising in various benign polyps are :
  * Endometrial polyp   Adenocarcinoma
  * Fibroid polyp   Sarcoma
  * Placental polyp   Choriocarcinoma.

* Characteristic features in Vulval CIN are "3P" as,
  * Pruritus
  * Pigmented area
  * Papule

Endometrial lesions

* The permalignant lesions of endometrium are endometrial hyperplasia of following varieties :
  1. Cystic hyperplasia.
  2. Adenomatous hyperplasia.
  3. Atypical hyperplasia.
  4. Carcinoma-in-situ.

Carcinoma Vulva

* Most common (MC \) type is well diffrentiated Sq. cell carcinoma.
* MC site of CAvulva is laboum Najus (second MC site = Clitoris).
* MC part of labium majus involved in Sq. cell Ca of vulva is anterior two-third
* MC mode of spread is through lymphatics
* MC type of lymphatic spread is by embolisation.
* MC symptoms is pruritus vulvae
* MC lymph node involved is inguinal
* MC pelvic lymph node involved is obturator.

Carcinoma vagina

* MC Malignancy of vagina is metastatic carcinoma.
* MC source of metastasis in vagina is Ca-cervix.
* Mc type of Primary carcinoma of vagina :
  1. Naked eye   Ulcerative type
  2. Histopathologically   Sq. cell C of vagina is upper third of posterior vaginal wall.
* MC site of Adenocarcinoma of vagina (due to intrauterine exposure to DES) is upper anterior vaginal wall.

CARCINOMA CERVIX

* MC cancer in women in most of the developing countries including India.
* MC site of involvement is squamocolumnar junction (ectocervix).
* MC cancer of Endocervical canal is Sq. cell. carcinoma (Not Adenocarcinoma as believed previously)
* MC organ involved in direct spread from sq. cell Ca of cervix is

vagina.

* MC organ in direct spread from Adenocarcinoma of cervix is body of uterus.

* **Risk Factors :**

   (i)   Early sexual activity

   (ii) Promiscuity

   (iii) Frequent intercourse

   (iv) Multiplicity of sexual partners

   (v)   Lower socio-economic classes.

   (vi) Viral infection   Herpes simplex type -2.

                                    Human papilloma virus type-16, 18, 31, 33.

   (vii) Heavy smoking.

   (viii) Women afflicted with AIDS.

   (ix) Sexually transmitted diseases.

   (x)   Young girls exposed to DES in utero (DES=Diethylstilbestrol).

   (xi) Early age at first intercourse.

   (xii) Early first pregnancy.

   (xiii)   Cervical dysplasia & carcinoma-in-situ.

   (xiv)   Too many births/too frequent birth.

* MC **mode of spread** of CA cervix is by lymphatics.

* Earliest lymphatic spread is to parametrial (paracervical) lymph nodes.

* MC site of distant nodal metastasis is supraclavicular lymph nodes.

* MC **cause of death** in CA cervix is uraemia.

* Least common mode of spread in CA cervix is hematogenous.

* MC organ involved due to hematogenous spread in Ca cervix is Lung.

* Earliest symptom in Exophytic growth & overall earliest symptoms is intermenstrual or postcoital bleeding.

* Most prominent feature in Endophytic growth is offensive vaginal discharge.

* Most important sign of CA cervix is friability.

ENDOMETRIAL CARCINOMA

* MC female genital malignancy in developed countries (In India CA Cervix is the MC genital malignancy in female).

* MC type is adenocarcinoma (Endrometroid).

* MC site in uterus is fundus.

* MC mode of spread is through Lymphatics.

* MC symptoms is postmenopausal bleeding.
* MC site of local recurrence following hysterectomy is vaginal vault.
* **Risk factors :**
  * Older age (usually postmenopausal)
  * Low parity (usually nullipara)
  * Early menarche
  * Late menopause
  * Unmarried
  * Corpus cancer syndrome (consists of Obesity, Hypertension and Diabetes mellitus)
  * Unopposed oestrogen stimulation due to
    * functioning ovarian tumor (Granulosa cell tumor)
    * polycystic ovarian syndrome (Stein-Leventhal syndrome)
    * oestrogen replaement therapy in post menopausal women.
  * Fibroid
  * Atypical complex endometrial hyperplasia
  * Diet rich in fat.
  * Radiation menopause
  * Familial.
  * MC site of metastasis is lung.
  * Sarcoma in fibroid has a better prognosis

CARCINOMA FALLOPIAN TUBE

* MC carcinoma of F. tube is metastatic carcinoma (secondaries).
* MC source of secondary in fallopian tube is ovary or uterus.
* MC mode of spread of secondary carcinoma is lymphatic permeation (not direct extension).
* MC primary carcinoma of fallopian tube is adenocarcinoma. MC site of adenocarcinoma is ampullary part.
* MC structure involved in adenocarcinoma of tube is tubal mucosa.
* MC earliest symptoms is watery vaginal discharge.
* Mostly unilaterl (80%)
* MC site fo metastasis of adenocarcinoma is omentum & peritoneum

MALIGNANT OVARIAN TUMORS

* Ranks third amongst gynecologic cancers.
* Accounts for 5% of all gynecological cancers in India.
* Mc cause of **death due to gynecological cancers** is ovarian carcinoma.

* MC ovarian cancer is papillary serous cystadenocarcinoma.
* Second MC ovarian cancer is endometroid carcinma.
* MC ovarian cancer in women under the age of 20 is dysgerminoma.
* MC hormonally active ovarian tumor is granulosa-theca cell tumors.
* More common amongst nulliparous

Clinical Associations :
* Nulliparity
* Cosmetic talc contaminated with asbestos
* Infertility
* Marked premenstrual tension
* Abnormal breast swelling
* Marked dysmenorrhoea
* Pelvic irradiation, and
* History of rubella & mumps.
* In postmenopausal patient with a pelvic mass, a amrkedly elevated serum CA-125 level (>95 U/mL) distinguishes malignant from benign ovarian epithelial tumor.
* Detection of malignant cells from the ascitic fluid sample when combined with presence of a pelvic mass almost confirms ovarian malignancy.
* Recently, most commonly employed mode of radiotherapy in Ca ovary is "moving strip feild technique".
* MC radioactive isotope used for intraperitoneal instillation in Ca ovary is radioactive phosphorous (32P) Othr is Chromic phosphate.

Dysgerminoma :
* MC malignant germ cell tumor (MC germ cell tumor is benign cystic teratoma)
* Only germ cell tumor in which the opposite ovary may be involved is dysgerminoma.
* Lymphocyte & giant cells are always found amongst tumor cells.
* MC site of metastasis is reroperitoneal lymph nodes.
* Schiller-Duval bodies are pathognomonic,
* Tumor markers are :
    * Alpha fetoprotein (AFP) - Serum value > 20 µg/mL
    * Alpha-1-antitrypsin
* Most important feature differentiating yolk sac tumor from other germ cell tumors is presence of pelvic pain.

* Responsible for on "Indian summer" state of the patient is granules cell tumor.
* Earliest site of metastasis in granulosa cell tumor is opposite ovary.
* MC site of primary in secondaries in ovary is GIT (pylorus, colon, & rarely small bowel).
* CA of uterus is 10 times more likely to metastasize to the ovary than that of cervix.
* Histologically, signet-ring cells are characteristic.
* MC primary site is stomach.
* Purplish nodular hemorrhagic metastasis into lower third of the vagina or around the vaginal orrifice is characteristic & pathognomonic of choriocarcinoma.
* Criteria for high risk metastatic gestational trophoblastic disease (GES):
  1. The duration of disease is longer than 4 months.
  2. There are liver & brain metastasis.
  3. The β HCG titer is > 100,000 mlU/mL
  4. It follows a full-term pregnancy
  5. Previous treatment with chemotherapy.

PEDIATRIC ONCOLOGY

WILMS TUMOR

* Also called **Nephroblastoma.**
* Most common cancer of kidney in children.
* Most common abdominal malignancy in children
* Most common site of haematogenous metastasis is lungs.
* Most important prognostic factor is its Histological type.
* Most significant associated anomalies constitutes 'WAGR' syndrome i.e. Wilm's Tumor, Aniridia, Genito Urinary anomalies (especially Horse shoe kidney) and mental Retardation.
* Classical triad of symptoms is :
  * Lump
  * Fever
  * Haematuria
* **'Egg-shell pattern'** periheral calcification is characteristic in plain X-ray abdomen, but it is found only in 10% cases.
* **Surgery** is the cornerstone in Wilms' tumor therapy.

NEUROBLASTOMA

* Highly malignant tumor of neural crest that form sympathetic ganglia and adrenal medulla.
* Most common solid malignant tumor of infancy after brain tumor.
* Most common site is adrenal medulla.
* Most common age group is below 2 years.
* Histopathology shows presence of neuroblast, which is a small round cell with large nucleus and scanty cytoplasm. **Rossette formation** is an important finding.
* **Dancing eye syndrome** (opsomyoclonus and nystagmus), a feature of cerebellar ataxia, sometime may be present in neuroblastoma
* X-ray abdomen may show **stippled calcification.**
* Most common site of metastasis in neuroblastoma in infant is **Liver.** Most common site of metastasis in older children is Bone.
* Most common site of bony metastasis is skull and diaphysis of distal femur and humerus.
* Most accurate method of biochemic diagnosis of neuroblastoma is determination of all catecholamines and their metabolites in a 24 hours urine collection.
* VMA (Vanillyl mandelic acid) and HVA (Homovanillic acid) are 2 important metabolites of catecholamines found in urine in cases of neuroblastoma.

RHABDOMYOSARCOMA

* Rhabdomyosarcoma can occur in any organ except brain. Most common site in male is bladder or prostate.
* Most common site in female is vagina.
* ost common site is ovary or testis.
* Most common site in **neonates** is the **sarcrococcygeal area.**
* It is malignant neoplasm of lymphoid tissue
* MC malignant lymphoma is Hodgkin's lymphoma.
* Most common (50%) site of lymphnode involvement in Hodgkin's lymphoma is cervical or supraclavicular. Most common (70%) group of lymphnode involvement in neck is superficial group.
* The term 'E' is used for presence of localised involvement of extralymphatic sites such as lung, pericardium bone (but not bone marrow) in Hodgkin's lymphoma.
* **Gallium scintigraphy** is useful in cetecting early recurrences and response to treatment.

* Most active new drug in NHL is **Fludarabine.**
* **Radiation** exposure increases the risk of developing:
  * CML   * AML   * ALL   * But not CLL and hairy cell Leukemia.
* Most patients with preleukemia and myelodysplastic syndrome never develops AML but the most comon cause of death in them is bone marrow failure.
* Smoldering AML is a type of leukemia in which the diagnostic features of acute leukemia are present but the disease has a **subacute course.**

Pathology

* The leukemic cells expansion follows a **Gompertzian growth curve.**
* **Auer rods** are diagnostic of AML and is found in only 10-20 patients of AML particularly in M3 type.
* M5 subtype of AML is most likely to involve extramedullary tissues.
* Tdt (deoxynucleotidyl transferase), a nuclear enzyme terminal, is found only in 20% AML-cells, whereas it is present in 90% of leukemic lymphoblasts.
* Acute leukemias of both lineages often express CD-34.
* Most myeloid leukemias express CD-33.
* Fever is the commonest (60% cases) symptom of acute leukemia. Common organisms causing infection are gram negative bacteria gram positive cocci and candida.
* Hepatosplenomegaly is the commonest sign in acute leukemia and is more common in ALL than AML.
* Commonest metabolic complications in acute leukemia are hyponatremia and hypokalemia
* Most anticancer drugs used in treatment of acute leukemia are to capable of 3-5 log cell kill and eliminates 99.9 to 99.999 percent of leukemic cells.
* Chronic lymphocytic leukemia is a neoplasm of activatd B lymphocytes.
* Most common type of leukemia is CLL.
* Commonly associated with trisomy-12.
* Dual expression of B-cell antigen and T-cell antigen on the CLL-cells are diagnostic.
* CLL cells have Fc receptors and CD-21.
* CLL may evolve into an aggressive lymphocyte lymphoma, known as **Richter's syndrome.**

* **Most commonly** used drug for CLL is chlorambucil.
* Drug useful in Packed syndrome is glucocorticoids.

Hairy cell leukemia

* **Hairy cell** are 15-20 μ in diameter and has an eccentrically.
* **Hairs** (cytoplasmic projections) in Hairy cell leukemia are bes seen by phase microscopy.

CML

* **Most common** complain in CML is **left upper abdomen** discomfort.
* **Most common** physical sign is **splenomegaly.**
* Neutrophil alkaline phosphatases is low or zero.
* **Cytogenetic study** is confirmatory in CML.
* Most common cause of death in juvenile CML is infection or organ failure.
* Drug of choice for chronic phase CML is hydroxyurea.
* MC primary malignant tumor of the bone.
* It is the malignant proliferation of plasma cells, derived from a single clone (Monoclonal gammopathy).
* MC symptom is bone pain, which is precipitated by movement.
* MC cause of persistent pain in a patient with multiple myeloma is pathological bone fracture.
* MC site of Bone lesions in multiple myeloma is vertebral column.
* MC site of localised palpable bone lesion is skull.
* Second MC clinical problem (next to bone pain) in patient with multiple myeloma is susceptibility to bacterial infections.
* MC pathogens involved in infections in patient with multiple myeloma are,

1. In Lung ->
   * Streptococcus pneumoniae (Pneumococcus) -> most pathogenic.
   * Staph. aureus and
   * Klebsiella pneumoniae.
2. In urinary tract -> E. coli & other gram (-ve) bacteria.

* MC cause of renal failure in multiple myeloma is hypercalcemia.
* Most consistent pathology of renal failure in multiple myeloma is tubular damage due to excreted light chains. the earliest manifestation of this tubular damage is the **Adult Fanconi syndrome** (type 2 renal tubular acidosis).
* **Carpal tunnel syndrome** may occur due to infiltration of peripheral nerves by **amyloid materials.**

* M-component is the complete immunoglobulin molecule secreted by the plasma cells in multiple myeloma
* Bence Jones Proteins are low molecular weight light chain either K or d* (produced by plasma cells in multiple myeloma) **excreted in urine.**
* Osteoclast activating factors are,
  * IL-1.
  * TNF-a*
  * Lymphotoxin

DO YOU KNOW

* Excluding skin cancers, MC malignancy worldwide is gastric cancer.
* MC malignant tumour of spleen is angiosarcoma.
* MC lymphoma is Hodgkin's lymphoma.
* MC renal manifestation o neoplastic disease is nephrotic syndrome.
* MC primay tumour which gives secondary to penis is bladder carcinoma.
* MC foramen magnum tumour is meningioma.
* MC cause of intrameduallary metastasis of spinal cord is bronchogenic carcinoma.
* MC neoplastic cause of anosmia is meningioma of the inferior frontal region.
* MC solid tumour associated with myelodysplastic syndrome is carcinoma breast.
* Most sensitive technique to detect malignant cell in Non-Hodgkin's lymphoma is PCR (polymerase chain reaction).
* MC cause od death in cutaneous T. Cell lymphoma is infection.
* MC malignancy in Ataxia-Telengiectasia is lymphoma.
* MC presentation of Kaposi's sarcoma in AIDS patient is raised macule.
* MC lymphoma in AIDS is diffuse histiocytic (immunoblastic) lymphoma.
* MC extranodal site for lymphoma in AIDS is CNS (2nd most common extraodal side is GIT).
* MC D/D of CNS lymphoma in AIDS is cerebral toxoplasmosis.
* MC malignancy associated with widespread systemic vascultis (classical PAN) is hairy cell leukemia.
* MC paraneoplastic neuropathy is sensorimotor neuropathy.
* MC secondary cause of Hypertrophic osteoarthropathy is bronchogenic carcinoma.
* MC symptom of carcinoid syndrome is flushing.
* MC malignancy associated with Erythroderma is cutaneous T-cell lymphoma (CTCL).

* Most useful diagnostic aid for "carcinoma-in-situ" of cervix is cone biopsy.
* The earliest symptom of invasive carcinoma cervix is post coital bleeding.
* "Reinke crystals" are seen in Hilus cell tumour of the ovary and also in arrhenoblastoma.
* Modified Basset's operation is done for carcinoma vulva.
* OVarian tumor most commonly associated with Steinleventhal syndrome is Dermoid.
* The MC positins for beginning of neoplasia of the cervix are 6 O'clock and 12 O' clock.
* "Coffee bean cells" are seen in Brenner tumour.
* MC anticancer drug causing transient urinary incontinence/urinary retentin is **Vincristine.**
* Cancer, the course of which is accelerated during pregnancy is **Breast cancers** (due to high estrogen level).
* Paraneoplastic **opsoclonus** is seen in :
  a. Neuroblastoma (in children)
  b. Carcinoma of ovary, lungs breast (in adults).
* Paraneoplastic opsoclonus is associated with the presence of following **antibodies** in the blood and spinal fluid :
  a. Anti-purkinje cell
  b. Anti anti-RHI
* MC cancer of gastroinestinal tract in India is CArcinoma esophagus (Ref Med. Guzzet, FEb. 1995, India).
* Second MC cancer of GIT in India is CA. rectum.
* Franz's tumour is papillary cystic neolasm of the pancreas.
* **Bazex' syndrome** is a distinctive paraneoplastic eruption associated with sq. cell CA of ,
  * Oropharynx
  * Tracheobronchial tree
  * Esophagus
* MC solid tumour of the **omentum** is metastatic carcinoma (secondaries)
* MC primary malignant tumour of omentum is leiomyosarcoma and hemangiopericytoma.
* MC benign mesenteric mass is **chylous** or **lymphati cysts.**
* MC site for the mesenteric tumor is, **mesentry of ileum.**
* MC tumour of retroperitoneum is malignant tumours.

* MC benign tumour of retroperitoneum is **lipoma.**
* MC malignant retroperitoneal tumour is **malignant lymphoma** or **lymphosarcoma.**
* Malignant retroperitoneal tumours having best prognosis are neuroblastoma and liposarcoma.
* MC soft-tissue swelling of hand is **ganlgion.**
* MC cause of superior venacava obstruction is **bronchogenic carcinoma** invading the mediastinum.
* MC bone tumour of hand is **enchondroma.**
* Alkylating agent of choice in the treatment of Hodgkin's disease is **mechlorethamine.**
* Anticancer drug discovered in India is **TAXOL.**
* MC tumour associated with tuberous sclerosis is **cardiac rhabdomyoma.**
* MC malignancy associated with tricholemmomas (an adnexal tumour) is CA. breast.
* Linear accelerator produces **photon** and **electron.**
* MC tumour associated with Torre's syndrome is multiple sebaceous adenoma (CA. colon is MC internal malignancy associated with Torre's syndrome).
* MC malignancy associated with sweet's syndrome is acute nonlymphocytic leukemia.
* Pseudo-Kaposi's sarcoma (**acral angiodermatitis**) is the parple papules on the lower extremities due to congenital or acquired A-V fistual (resembling Kaposi's sarcoma clinicaly and histologically).
* MC site of angiosarcoma is **scalp and face.**
* MC primary malignancy which gives rise to cutaneous metastasis is lung carcinoma (male) and **breast carcinoma** (female).
* **Gompertzian growth of cancer cells** tells that, as a tumour mass increases, the time required to double the tumour's volume also increases.
* "Rought rule of ten" is associated with Pheochromocytoma.
* MC brain tumour which leads to development of dementia is **meningioma of frontal lobe.**
* MC extracranial neoplasm related with the increased risk for organic mental disorder is **carcinoma pancreas.**
* Antineoplastic drug which can be used to produce fetal haemoglobin for the treatment of sickle cell anemia or thalassemia is **hydroxyurea.**
* **CEA** is used as tumour marker in cancers of :

  —Colon

  —Stomach

—Lungs

—Breast

—Pancreas.

* **AFP** is used as tumour marker in cancers of :

—Liver

—GIT

—Testicular cancers.

* **'Buschke Lowenstein Tumor'** is a massive venereal wart.

* **Osteolytic** bone metastasis are found in cancers of :

—Thyroid

—Kidney

—Colon and rectum

—Breast

* **Osteoblastic** bone metastasis are found in cancers of :

—Prostate

—Breast

—Malignant carcinoid tumour

—Hodgkin's disease

* Cancers causing **lymphedema** includes :

—CA. prostate

—CA. breast

* Single most important feature distinguishing benign from malignant tumour is metastasis.

* Anticancer drug causing **hemolysis in G6PD deficiency** doxorubicin.

* TOC in desmoid tumor is **surgery.**

     * Other Tt includes.

         * Radiotherapy

         * Tamoxifen

         * Prostaglandin inhibitors.

* MC site for superficial erythmatous basal cell cancer (**"body basal"**) is trunk.

* Amount of **normal skin-margin** included in surgical excision of skin cancer is,

     * Basal cell carcinoma   3 mm.

     * Sq cell carcinoma   1 cm.

     * Malignant melanoma   3 cm.

* MC metastatic tumors associated with **Intracerebral hemorrhage,** include.
  * Choriocarcinoma
  * Malignant melanoma.
  * Renal cell carcinoma
  * Bronchogenic carcinoma
* MC type of NHL, which presents with prominent **mediastinal mass** is lymphoblastic lymphoma.
* MC cancer presenting with peripheral blood manifestatin of hyposplenism in the presence of splenomegaly (or, normal sized spleen) is **primay splenic angiosarcoma.**
* Endodermal sinus tumor of ovary is also known as teilum tumor.

METAPLASIA VERSUS DYSPLASIA

	Feature	Metaplasia	Dysplasia
1.	Definition	Adaptive substitution of one type of adult cell type by another well differentiated adult cell type	No substitution of cells as in metaplasia
2.	Development of cells	Not deranged	Deranged
3.	Adaptation	An adaptive process	Not adaptive
4.	Association with hyperplasia	None	Associations present
5.	Cellular changes	No changes in : — cell size and shape — nucleus — mitotic figures — abundant mitotic figures	Changes present are : — pleomorphism — changes in nucleus — (Hyperchromatic)
6.	Site	Occurs in epithelial and mesenchymal cells	Occurs only in epithelial cells
7.	Conversion to Neoplasia	Lesser	More

DYSPLASIA VERSUS ANAPLASIA

	Feature	Dysplasia	Anaplasia
1.	Definition	A disturbance in growth which is usually considered to be pre-malignant	It is a property of malignancy which consists of undifferentation of cells
2.	Development of cells	Deranged	No differentiation of cells
3.	Reversibility	Reversible	Irreversible

4.	Mitosis	Normal	Abnormal in number
5.	Giant cells	Absent	Present
6.	Necrosis necrosis	Absent	Tumour cells may undergo
7.	Polarity of cells	Present	Lost
8.	Conversion to neoplasia	Can give rise to neoplasia	Anaplasia is itself a property of neoplasia
9.	Features of Anaplasia	Absent	

PARANEOPLASTIC SYNDROMES

Clinical Syndrome Endocrinopathies	Major Forms of Underlying Cancer	Causal Mechanism
Cushing's syndrome	Bronchogenic carcinoma Malignant thymoma Pancreatic carcinoma	Adrenocorticotropin or ACTH-like substance
Hyponatremia	Bronchogenic carcinoma Intracranial neoplasma	Antidiuretic hormone or ADH-like substance
Hypercalcemia	Bronchogenic carcinoma Bronchogenic squamous carcinoma, Renal carcinoma Endometrial carcinoma	Parathromone or PTH-like substance ?prostaglandins, uncertain origin
Hyperthyroidism	Blood dyscrasia Bronchogenic carcinoma Prostatic carcinoma	Thyroid-stimulating hormone or TSH-like substance
Hypoglycemia	Fibrosarcoma Hepatocellular carcinoma	Insulin or insulin-like substance
Carcinoid syndrome	Bronchial adenoma (carcinoid) Pancreatic carcinoma Gastric carcinoma	Serotonin, bradykinin, ?histamine
Polycythemia	Renal carcinoma Cerebellar hemangioma Hepatocellular carcinoma	Erythropoietin
Nerve and muscle syndromes		
Myasthenia	Bronchogenic carcinoma Breast carcinoma	?Immunologic, ?toxic
Disorder of the central and peripheral nervous systems *Dermatologic disorders*		
Acanthosis nigricans	Gastric carcinoma Lung carcinoma Uterine carcinoma	?Immunologic, ?toxic
Dermatomyositis	Bronchogenic, breast carcinoma	?Immunologic, ?toxic
Osseous, articular, and soft tissue changes		
Hypertrophic osteoarthropathy and clubbing of the fingers	Bronchogenic carcinoma	Unknown
Vascular and hematologic changes		
Venous thrombosis (Trousseau's phenomenon)	Pancreatic carcinoma Bronchogenic carcinoma Other cancers	?Hypercoagulability
Marantic endocarditis (nonbacterial thrombotic vegetations)	Advanced cancers	?Hypercoagulability
Anemia	Thymic neoplasms	Unknown
Leukemoid reaction	Thymic neoplasms	Unknown

COMMON TUMOR-DERIVED PRODUCTS

Biochemically Monitored

Tumor-derived products	Associated Neoplasm
Oncofetal antigens	
Carcinoembryonic antigen (CEA)	Carcinoma of colon, rectum, pancreas, liver, bron chus, others
Alpha-fetoprotein (AFP)	Carcinoma of liver, gonads, stomach, pancreas, others
Hormones	
Chorionic gonadotropin	Choricarcinoma, hydatidiform mole
Calcitonin	Carcinoma of lung or breast, medullary carcinoma of the thyroid
Prostaglandins	Carcinoma of lung or breast
Relevant hormones	Tumors of endocrine glands
Ectopic hormones	Paraneoplastic syndromes
Enzymes	
Acid phsophatase	Carcinoma of prostate
Alkaline phosphatase	Carcinoma of liver, osteogenic sarcoma

APUD CELLS, APUDOMAS, AND ECTOPIC POLYPEPTIDE HORMONES PRODUCED BY APUDOMAS

Cell	Putative Tumor	Hormone
Hypothalamic neurosecretory	Non identified	
Pinealocyte	Pinealoma	Unknown
Adenohypophyseal	Pituitary adenoma	Unknown
Autonomic neuron	Neurocytoma	ACTH; vasoactive intestinal peptide (VIP)
Chromaffin	Pheochromocytoma calcitonin (CT); insulin	ACTH; follicle-stimulating hormone;
Carotid-body and other paraganglion cells	Paraganglioma; chemodectoma	ACTH; CT
Thyroid C	Meduallary carcinoma of thyroid	ACTH; insulin
Bronchial Kulchitsky	Bronchial carcinoid; oat cell carcinoma	ACTH; ADH; CT glucagon; insulin; growth hormone; prolactin
Gastrointestinal endocrine	Intestinal carcinoid	ACTH; ADH
Pancreatic islet	Islet cell tumor	ACTH; ADH; VIP
Melanocyte	Melanoma	ACTH; gastrin Present characteristically

HEREDITARY CANCEROUS AND PRECANCEROUS DISORDERS

Disorder	Predominant Tumors
Autosomal Dominant Inheritance	
Retinoblastoma	Retinoblastoma, sarcoma orbital (following radiation) and at remote sites
Neurofibromatosis	Neurogenic sarcoma, acoustic neuroma, pheochromocytoma
Familial polyposis coli	Colonic cancer, adenomatous polyps
Gardner's syndrome	Colonic cancer, adenomatous polyps
Peutz-Jegher's syndrome	Controversial whether predisposes to colonic cancer.
Hereditary multiple endocrine neoplasia syndrome— type I (MEN I)	Tumors of the pituitary gland, parathyroid gland, and pancreatic islet cells
Multiple endocrine neoplasia syndrome—type II (MEN II)	Medullary carcinoma of the thyroid, pheochromocytoma and parathyroid disease
Cutaneous malignant melanoma	Cutaneous malignant melanoma, other cancers
Von Hippel-Lindau's syndrome	Hemangioblastoma of cerebellum, hypernephroma, and pheochromocytoma
Kaposi's syndrome	Sarcoma, lymphoma
Cancer-family syndrome	Adenocarcinomas (primarily of the colon and endometrium)
Breast cancer in association with other malignant neoplasms	Breast cancer, sarcoma, leukemia, and brain tumor
Autosomal Recessive Inheritance	
Xeroderma pigmentosum	Basal and squamous cell carcinoma of skin, malignant melanoma
Fanconi's anemia	Leukemia and lymphoma
Bloom's syndrome	Acute leukemia
Ataxia telangiectasia	Acute leukemia, lymphoma and possibly gastric cancer
Turcot's syndrome	Colonic polyps, cancer and brain tumors

CLINICAL FEATURES OF BENIGN AND MALIGNANT ULCERS

		Benign Ulcer	Malignant Ulcer
1.	Age of patient	Tends to occur in younger individuals	Tends to occur in older individuals
2.	Duration of symptoms	Varies from weeks to many years	Varies from weeks to months but rarely for years
3.	Sex	Marked male preponderance	Slight male preponderance
4.	Gastric acidity	May be normal or increased-anacidity rare	Usually normal levels but can be totally absent

5.	Location of lesion	Usually lesser curvature of pyloric or prepyloric region-however, may be on greater curvature or anterior or posterior wall.	Greater curvature of pyloric and prepyloric regions-however, may on lesser curvature in other sites in stomach
6.	Size of lesion	Usually is less than 2 cm in diameter and rarely over 4 cm	Usually greater than 4 cm in diameter but may be smaller
7.	Response to medical therapy	Usually shows prompt evidence of healing on adequate treatment	May respond to medical therapy but usually is refractory
8.	X-ray	Demonstrates a small punched-out niche without involvement of surrounding wall	Demonstrates defect with irregular or heaped-up margins and possible involvement of surrounding wall and mucosa

GENETIC SYNDROMES ASSOCIATED WITH MULTIPLE PRIMARY TUMOURS

	Genetic syndrome	Nervous tissue Neoplasm	Associated Neoplasms
1.	Cowdens disease (multiple hamartoma syndrome)	Meningioma	Papillomas of lip and mouth. Cancer of breast. Adenoma and carcinoma of thyroid. Lipoma, Polyps cysts of bone and liser.
2.	Nevoid basal cell Carcinoma syndrome	Medulloblastoma	Basal cell carcinomas Tumours of ovaries
3.	Sipples syndrome (Multiple endocrine adenoatosis II) Brain tumour	Phaeochromocytoma Neurofibromas Submucosal neuromas neoplams	Medullary thyroid carcinoma Parathyroid
4.	Turcot's syndrome	Brain tumour	Polyposis coli
5.	Werner's syndrome (Multiple Endocrine (Adenomatosis I)	Anterior Pituitary	Parathyroid Pancreatic islet cells, thyroid, adrneal cortex, carcinod (bronchus and intestine)

IMPORTANT PREMALIGNANT LESION

1. Chronic atrophic gastritis of pernicious anemia

2. Solar keratosis

3. Child breakage syndrome

4. Chronic ulcerative colitis

5. Leukoplakia   —oral cavity

                           —vulva & penis

6. Bowen's disease of skin/penis

7. Erythroplasia of Querat

8.   Multiple polyposis
9.   Pseudo epitheliomatous hyperplasia
10.   Kraurosis vulvae
11.   Cirrhosis of liver
12.   Haemochromatosis
13.   Chronic cervicitis

FEW BORDERLINE MALIGNANCY

1.   Thyroid adenoma.   4.   Mycosis fungoides
2.   Bronchial adenoma   5.   Osteoclastoma.
3.   Paget's disease of breast/bone.

LOCALLY MALIGNANT TUMOUR

1.   Basal cell carinoma   3.   Solitary plasmacytoma.
2.   Osteoclastoma.

PREGNANCY TUMOUR

1.   Angiogranuloma of the gingiva   2.   Granuloma gravidarum.

TUMOR MARKERS

	Markers	Levels Increase in (Cancers)
1.	**Hormones**	
	i) Human Chorionic Gonadotropin (HCG)	Non-seminomatous tumours, Trophoblastic tumours
	ii) Calcitonin	Medullary carcinoma thyroid
	iii) Catecholamines	Pheochromocytoma
2.	**Oncofetal Antigens**	
	i) Alfa-Fetoprotein	Non-seminomatous germ cell testicular tumours, hepatocellular Ca
	ii) Carcinoembryonic Antigen (CEA)	Carcinoma G.I.T. Breast
3.	**Isoenzymes**	
	i) Prostatic Acid Phosphatase	Ca Prostate
	ii) Neurone Specific Enolase	Small cell Ca of Lung, neuroblastoma
4.	**Specific Proteins**	
	i) Immunoglobulins	Multiple Myeloma
	ii) Prostate-Specific Antigen	Ca Prostate
	iii) Various polypeptide	Neuroendocrine tumors (carcinoid/Islet cell)

iv) Coagulation factor VIII   Angiosarcoma
related antigen

v) Myoglobin, muscle opacification   Melanomas, varsous
and myosin desmin

vi) 5-100 protein   Other cell types (Schwann cells, chondro-
cytes)

5.   **Mucins, etc,**
    i)   CA-125   Ca Ovary
    ii)   CA-19-9   Ca Colon, pancreas
    iii)   CA-15-3   Ca breast

6.   **Intermediate filaments**
    i)   Cytokeratin   —All carcinomas.
    ii)   Vimentin   Mesenchymal lesions sarcomas, also in
    epithelial tumors.
    iii)   Neuro filament   All neuronal & neuroendocrine cells
    iv)   Glial fibrillary acidic   Non neuronal brain tissue
    protein (GFAP)
    v)   Desmin   Muscle cells.

7.   **Other general markers**
    i)   Leukocyte common antigen (LCA)   Lymphomas

CHEMICALS RECOGNIZED AS CARCINOGENS IN HUMANS

Chemical	*Sites of Cancers*
Chemical Mixtures	
Soots, tars, oils	Skin lungs
Cigarette smoke and tars	Lungs, bladder
Industrial Chemicals	
2-Naphthylamine	Urinary bladder
Benzidine	Urinary bladder
4-Aminobiphenyl	Urinary bladder
Chloromethyl, ethyl ether	Lungs
Nickel compounds	Lungs, nasal sinuses
Chromium compounds	Lungs
Asbestos	Lungs, pleura
Arsenic compounds	Skin, lungs
Vinyl chloride	Liver
Drugs	
N, N-bis (2 chloroethyl)-2	Urinary bladder
Diethylstibestrol	Vagina
Phenacetin	Renal pelvis
Oral contraceptives	Benign hepatomas naphthylamine
Naturally Occurring Compounds	
Aflatoxins	Liver
Betal nuts	Buccal mucosa

CLASSIFICATION OF THE LEUKEMIAS

Lymphocytic Acute (Lymphoblastic) (ALL)

L1   Small cells predominate but may vary, with some cells up to twice the diameter of the small lymphocytes. Nuclei are generally round and regular with occasional clefts. Nucleoli are often not visible. Cytoplasm is scanty. The cell population is homogeneous.

L2   Cells are heterogeneous in size and share in the features of both L1 and L3. Nuclei often show clefts. Nucleoli are often present.

L3   There is a homogenous population of large cells (3 to 4 times the diameter of small lymphocytes). Nuclei are round to oval with prominent nucleoli. Cytoplasm is abundant and deeply basophilic.

Chronic Lymphocytic (CLL).

Cells comprise a homogenous population of small mature lymphocytes, often associated with lymphocytic, well differentiated lymphoma.

Acute Myelocytic (Myeloblastic) (AML)

M1   Myeloblastic leukemia without maturation-cells are dominantly blasts without Auer rods or granules

M2   Myeloblastic leukemia with maturation-Many blasts but some maturation to promyelocytes or beyond.

M3   Hypergranular promyelocytic leukemia-Mostly promyelocytes with cytoplasm packed with peroxidase-positive granules. Many Auer rods.

M4   Myelomonocytic leukemia-Both myeloid and morocytic differentiation. Myeloid element resembles M2

M5   Monocytic leukemia-Both "monoblasts" and monocytes, the former having large round nuclei with lacy chromatin and prominent nucleoli. Diagnosis must be coafirmed by fluoride-inhibited esterase reaction.

M6.   Erythroleukemia-Erythropoietic elements comprise more than 50% of cells in marrow and have bizarre multilobate nuclei. May also be present in circulating blood, along with an admixture of myeloblasts and promyelocytes.

Chronic Myelocytic (CML)

Mostly neutrophils with scattered myelocytes and promyelocytes.

Acute Monocytic (included as M4, myelomonocytic leukemia)

Chronic Monocytic

Very uncommon. Mostly mature monocytes with scattered blasts. Some cells are peroxidase positive.

Special Rare Types

Histiocytic leukemia-May occur in histiocytic lymphoma.

Hairy-cell leukemia associated with leukemic reticuloendotheliosis-Of uncertain cell type. May be a B cell or possibly a histiocyte.

Leukemia associated with Sezary's syndrome. Thought to be of T-cell origin

Stem cell leukemia-Cells so immature as to be unidentifiable.

PRIMARY INTRACRANIAL NEOPLASMS*

Neuroepithelial	*Ectodermal*
Astrocytoma, grades I, II, II, and IV	Craniopharyngioma
Ependymomas	Pituitary adenomas
Oligodendrogliomas	
Medulloblastoma	*Congenital*
Pinealoma	Epidermoid
Papilloma of choroid plexus	Dermoid
Paraphyseal (colloid) cyst	
Neurilemoma	
Mesodermal	
Meningiomas	
Hemangioblastoma	
Chordoma	

* Neoplasms occurring with extreme rarity have been omitted from this classification, those tumors listed in the plural term occur with varying histological types and grades of differentiation.

ORIGINAL SOLVED MCQ's IN ONCOLOGY

GENERAL ASPECTS

1. **Which is not a precancerous lesion :**
   A. Leucoplakia
   B. Vesical papilloma
   C. Chronic cervictis
   D. Osteogenesis imperfecta

2. **The commonest site for lipoma to become malignant is :**
   A. Subcutaneous
   B. Retro-peritoneal
   C. Intramuscular
   D. Subaponeurotic

3. **The following are tumor markers except :**
   A. Albumin
   B. Thyroglobulin
   C. AFP
   D. CEA

4. **Epidermoid carcinoma of the following has best prognosis :**
   A. Lip
   B. Buccal mucosa
   C. Palate
   D. Brain

5. **The commonest retroperitoneal tumour is :**
   A. Lipoma
   B. Leiomyoma
   C. Hamartoma
   D. Fibroma

6. **Locally malignant tumor is :**
   A. Chondroma
   B. Chordoma
   C. Hamartoma
   D. Choristoma

7. **Increase in the size of an organ due to increase in the size of individual cells is :**
   A. Hyperplasia
   B. Dysplasia
   C. Hypetrophy
   D. Metaplasia

8. **Genetically determined tumours inlclude the following except :**
   A. Polyposis cell
   B. Retinoblastoma
   C. Multiple neurofibroma
   D. Neuroblastoma

9. **All of the following Ca are correctly matched with markers except :**
   A. Medullary-Thyrotropin
   B. Colon-CEA
   C. Testicular-HCG
   D. Hepatoma-AFP

Ans.	1. D	2. B	3. A	4. A	5. A	6. B
	7. C	8. D	9. C			

10. The content of myxoma is :
   A. Glycoprotein   B. Mucopolysacharide
   C. Glycogen   D. Fat

11. To differentiate benign and malignant stomach ulcer, best is :
   A. Cytology   B. Acid output
   C. Endoscopy and biopsy D. Barium meal

12. Kaposi's sarcoma arises from :
   A. Skin
   B. Fibrous tissue
   C. Connective tissue
   D. Capillaries and connective tissue

13. True about tumour cells is :
   A. Rate of growth is greater than normal cells
   B. Rate of multiplication decreases as size increases
   C. Rate of multiplication decreases as size decreases
   D. Rate of multiplication is not related to size

14. Exfoliative cytology is of special importance in   carcinoma :
   A. Lung   B. Cervix
   C. Kidney   D. Stomach

15. The most precise definition of a neoplasm is :
   A. Cancer   B. Carcinoma
   C. Tumor   D. Autonomous new growth

16. Which of the following is absolute proof of malig-   nancy of a tumor ?
   A. Invasion   B. Anaplasia
   C. Metastases   D. Rapid growth

17. A substance that will not produce cancer when acting alone but that will produce cancer when acting in conjunction with another substance is best described as a (n) :
   A. Carcinogen   B. Cocarcinogen
   C. Procarcinogen   D. Direct acting carcinogen

18. Leiomyoma is a tumour of :
   A. Smooth muscle cells   B. Fibroblasts
   C. Striated muscle cells D. Primitive mesenchyme

19. The most radioresistant tumour among the following is :
   A. Fibrosarcoma
   B. Embryonal carcinoma
   C. Squamous cell carcinoma
   D. Lymphosarcoma
   E. Lympho-epithelioma

Ans.	10. B	11. C	12. D	13. A	14. B	15. D
	16. C	17. B	18. A	19. A		

20. **Malignant cells are charactersised by :**
   A. A small nucleus
   B. A small nucelolus in relation to the nucelus
   C. A large nucleolus in relation to the nucleus
   D. Decreased nuclear chromatin
   E. Inter-cellular bridges

21. **A benign tumor is usually characterised by :**
   A. Pseudocapsule formed by compression of surroun-ding tissue
   B. Focal nuclear hyperchromatism
   C. Diffuse nuclear hyperchromatism
   D. Slow growth rate
   E. Immature cell population

22. **Inherited cancer syndrome consists of followingexcept :**
   A. Neurofibromatosis   B.   MEN
   C. Retinoblastoma   D.   Xeroderma pigmentosa

23. **Paramalignant effusion is seen in :**
   A. Hypoproteinemia
   B. Lymphatic block
   C. Malignancy related cachexia
   D. Hypocoagulability

24. **Which is not carcinogenic :**
   A. Benzpyrine   B.   Aniline dye
   C. Vitamin A   D.   Aflatoxin B1

25. **Which of the following feature differentiates carcinoma-in-situ from invasive carcinoma :**
   A. Pleomorphism
   B. Cartwheel appearance of nucleus
   C. Increased mitotic activity
   D. Basement membrane invasion

26. **With of the following is/are precancerous conditon(s)?**
   1. Intradermal naevus
   2. Polyposis coli
   3. Verrucus vulgaris
   4. Gastric intestinal metaplasia
   Select the correct answer :
   A. 1,2,3 and 4   B.   1 and 3
   C. 2 and 4   D.   3 alone

27. **Which of the following pairs of carcinogenic factorsand histological type of cancer are correctly matched ?**
   1. Solar radiation   Basal cell carcinoma
   2. Heredity   Retinoblastoma
   3. Herpes virus II   Carcinoma cervix

Ans.	20. C	21. D	22. D	23. B	24. C	25. D
	26. C	27. A				

Select the correct answer
A. 1, 2 and 3   B.   1 and 2
C. 1 and 3   D.   2 and 3

28. **Which of the following mechanisms are involved in the transformation of protooncogenes into oncogenes?**
1. Activation by point mutations
2. Activation by translocations
3. Activation by gene amplifications
Select the correct answer using the codes given below :
Codes :
A. 1,2 and 3   B.   1 and 2
C. 1 and 3   D.   2 and 3

29. **Consider the following statements :**
Grading of malignant neoplasm is based on the :
1. Extent and spread to adjacent structures
2. Degree of differentiation of tumour cells
3. Number of mitoses within the tumour
Of these statements
A. 1,2 and are correct   B.   1 and 2 are correct
C. 2 and 3 are correct   D.   1 and 3 are correct

30. **DNA probe analysis is of great value in the identifi- cation of gene in all of the following neoplasms except :**
A. Neuroblastoma   B.   Breast cancer
C. Lymphomas   D.   Gliomas

31. **Match List I (Markers) with List II (Malignancies) and select the correct answer using the codes given below the Lists :**

List I	List II
A. Alpha-foeto protein	1. Small cell carcinoma of lung
B. Human chorionic gonadotrophin	2. Hepatocellular carcinoma
C. Neuron-specific enolase	3. Carcinoma of colon
D. Carcinoma-embryonic antigen	4. Choriocarcinoma

Codes :

	A	B	C	D
A.	4	2	1	3
B.	4	2	3	1
C.	2	4	3	1
D.	2	4	1	3

Ans.	28. A	29. A	30. D	31. D

32. **Condition prone for malignancy :**
   A. Xeroderma pigmentosum   B. Cystic fibrosis
   C. Hamartomas   D. von Gierke's Disease

33. **All are tumour suppressor genes except:**
   A. Mad max gene   B. Retinoblastoma gene
   C. P53 gene   D. N - mic gene

34. **Teratomas the tumors that differentiate along which of the following germ layers :**
   A. Ectoderm and Endoderm
   B. Endoderm and Mesoderm
   C. Ectoderm, endoderm and Mesoderm
   D. Ectoderm and Mesoderm
   E. Mesoderm only

35. **In multiple myeloma - amyloid is :**
   A. AL   B. AA
   C. ATTR   D. $A\beta_2 m$

36. **Cancer cells derive energy via :**
   A. Fatty acid oxidation
   B. Glycolysis
   C. Oxidative phosphorylation
   D. Mitochondria

37. **The tumor suppressor gene present in head and neck tumors is :**
   A. P43   B. P53
   C. P63   D. P73

38. **Not a tumor marker :**
   A. Tartarate resistant alkaline phosphatase
   B. CEA
   C. AFP
   D. Alpha-1 antitrypsin

39. **To which of the following events the good outcome in Neuroblastoma is associated with ?**
   A. Diploidy   B. N-myc amplification
   C. Chromosome 1 p deletion D. Trk A expression

40. **The commonest site of oral cancer among Indian population is ?**
   A. Tongue   B. Floor of mouth
   C. Alveobuccal complex   D. Lip

41. **An exmple of a tumour suppressor gene is :**
   A. myc   B. fos
   C. ras   D. Rb

Ans.	32. A	33. A	34. C	35. A	36. B	37. B
	38. D	39. D	40. C	41. A		

42. Which one of the following is not used as a tumor marker in testicular tumors?

A. AFP

C. HCG

B. LDH

D. CEA

43. A simple bacterial test for mutagenic carcinogens is :

A. Ames test

C. Bacteriophage

B. Redox test

D. Gene splicing

44. Single pigmented naevi on the hand may be premalignant. They should be :

A. Left alone

C. Fulgurated

E. Excised

B. Cauterized

D. Irradiated

45. Maximum normal adult level of alpha fetoprotein is less than ——————— :

A. 10ng/ml

C. 14ng/ml

B. 12ng/ml

D. 16ng/ml

46. Hutchison's freckle is a type of :

A. Haemangioma

C. Melanoma

B. Fibroma

D. Lipoma

47. Raised level of carcinoma-embryonic antigen is seen in :

A. Ca.Breast

C. Ovarian Cancer

B. Lung Cancer

D. Ca. colon

48. Lesion most likely to undergo malignancy is :

A. Intrademal naevus

C. Actinic dermatitis

B. Junctional naevus

D. Dermal naevi

49. Mode of spread of Sarcoma is :

A. Lymphatics

C. Nerves

B. Blood vessels

D. Direct invasion

50. ↑ incidence with U.V. light exposure causes :

A. Basal Cell Ca

C. Adeno Ca

B. Sq. cell Ca

D. None of the above

51. Bowen's disease of the skin is :

A. A type of dermatitis

B. A tumour of sweat glands

C. A premallignent intradermal condition.

D. None of the above.

52. In internal organs, haemangioma is most commonly seen in :

A. Liver

C. Kidney

B. Spleen

D. Heart

Ans.	42. D	43. A	44. E	45. A	46. C	47. D
	48. D	49. B	50. A	51. C	52. A	

53. **Which of the following is not true about basal cell carcinoma :**
    A. Most common site is upper part of face
    B. Faster growing malignancy than Sq. cell carcinoma
    C. Lymphatic spread uncommon
    D. Prolonged exposure to sunlight is a predisposing factor

54. **The term "chemodectoma" denotes a tumour involving the :**
    A. Adrenal gland   B. Pituitary
    C. Carotid bodies   D. Spinal cord
    E. Heart

55. **Melanoma should be excised with a margin of :**
    A. 2 cm   B. 5 cm
    C. 7 cm   D. 10 cm
    E. None of the above

56. **Strawberry angioma in a child is treated by :**
    A. Masterly inactivity   B. Injection of sclerosants
    C. Injection of hot water   D. Excision and skin graftin

57. **The commonest malignancy in men over the age of sixty-five is :**
    A. Multiple myeloma
    B. Oropharyngeal carcinoma
    C. Prostatic carcinoma
    D. Carcinoma rectum

58. **Alpha feto protein levels are raised in all except :**
    A. Embryonic cell carcinoma
    B. Endodermal sinus tumour
    C. Hepatoma
    D. Fetus

59. **The term universal tumour refers to :**
    A. Adenoma   B. Papilloma
    C. Fibroma   D. Lipoma

60. **Squamous cell carcinoma can arise from:**
    A. Long standing venous ulcers
    B. Chronic lupus valgaris
    C. Rodent ulcer
    D. All of the above

61. **Carcinosarcoma is seen in :**
    A. Liver   B. Uterus
    C. Breast   D. Skin

62. **Prognosis in malignant melanoma is indicated by :**
    A. Depth of invasion   B. Giant cells
    C. Colour of lesion   D. Site of lesion

Ans.	53. B	54. C	55. B	56. A	57. C	58. B
	59. D	60. D	61. B	62. A		

63. **Malignant cell in Hodgkin's lymphoma is :**
A. Reed Sternberg cell   B. Lymphocytes
C. Histiocyte   D. Reticulum cells

64. **The TNM classification for malignancies is a :**
A. Clinical classification
B. Clinioradiological classification
C. Histological classification
D. Radiological classification

W65. **All of the following metastasize to lymph nodes in neck except :**
A. Ca tongue   B. Ca pharynx
C. Ca cheek   D. Ca vocal cords

66. **The malignant tumours that spread by predominantly by vascular permeation is :**
A. Carcinoma of the breast B. Lymphosarcoma
C. Renal cell carcinoma D. Basal cell carcinoma

67. **True about leukoplaqia :**
A. Is premalignant
B. Aspergillus infection
C. Gonorrhoea is a rare caus
D. Smoking is a rare cause

68. **Which of the following is premalignant :**
A. Angular stomatitis
B. Leukoplaqia vulva
C. Glandular hypertrophy of stomach
D. All of the above

69. **Margins of squamous cell carcinoma are :**
A. Inverted   B. Everted
C. Rolled   D. Undermined

70. **Keloid is common in :**
A. Dark people   B. Pregnancy
C. Tuberculosis   D. All of the above

71. **All of the following are benign tumors except :**
A. Chondroma   B. Chordoma
C. Synovioma   D. Neurolemmoma

72. **Ultimate difference in begning and malignant tumour is :**
A. Local infilteration   B. Metastasis
C. Mitotic Figures   D. Death

73. **Apudomas can arise from the following except:**
A. Pancreas   B. Skin
C. Intestine   D. Lymphnodes

Ans.	63. A	64. A	65. NONE	66. C	67. A	68. B
	69. B	70. A	71. B	72. B	73. D	

74. **Steriod therapy is useful in one of the following haemangioma :**
    A. Cavernous   B. Capillary
    C. Strawberry   D. Haemangiomas of adult

75. **A lustreless black lesion under the great toe nail of a 50 year old patient, noticed for three months is likely to be :**
    A. Sub-ungual haematoma   B. Glomus tumour
    C. Malignant melanoma   D. Chronic paronychia

76. **Secondaries are not seen in :**
    A. Breast   B. Brain
    C. Lung   D. Testis

77. **Neuroblastoma may arise at any of following sites except :**
    A. Posterior mediastinum   B. Adrenals
    C. Cervical region   D. Brain

78. **Which of the following neoplasms has a definite tendency to run in families?**
    A. Astrocytoma
    B. Carcinoma of the prostate
    C. Multiple adenomatous polyps of the colon
    D. Osteogenic sarcoma

79. **The treatment of a malignant melanoma should include all of the following except :**
    A. Wide excision of the tumour
    B. En bloc removal of the adjacent, involved lymph nodes
    C. Immediate excision of any enlarging lymph node in the postoperative period
    D. Postoperative radiotherapy to the surgical area and the adjacent lymph node

80. **Grossly visible venous invasion is a characteristic feature of carcinoma of the :**
    A. Breast   B. Colon
    C. Kidney   D. Ovary

81. **The following tumur has multicentric origin :**
    A. Basal cell carcinoma   B. Malignant melanoma
    C. Squamous cell carcinoma D. Lymphatic leukemia

82. **Regarding glomus tumour, which of the following is not true ?**
    A. It is a red/purple nodule under digital nail
    B. It is painless
    C. It resembles a naevus
    D. Histologically, it is angiomyoneuroma

Ans.	74. C	75. C	76. D	77. D	78. C	79. D
	80. C	81. D	82. B			

83. **Commonest cancer in males in india is of :**
    A. Bronchus   B. Stomatch
    C. Head and neck area   D. Urinary bladder

84. **In which of the following, metastasis disappears if primary is removed surgically :**
    A. Colon   B. Kidney
    C. Melanoma   D. Lung

85. **Familial tendency is seen in following except :**
    A. Ca breast   B. Ca stomach
    C. Ca colon   D. Ca larynx

86. **Metastatic carcinomatous lymph nodes are :**
    A. Soft and matted   B. Soft and fluctuant
    C. Very hard   D. None of the above

87. **Commenest benign soft tumor is :**
    A. Lipoma   B. Leiomyoma
    C. Hamartoma   D. Fibroma

88. **Commonest site of lymphangiosarcoma is :**
    A. Retroperitoneum
    B. Post mastectomy edema of arm
    C. Liver
    D. Spleen

89. **Which is not a neoplasm :**
    A. Pott's puffy tumour   B. Sarcoma
    C. Carcinoma   D. Papilloma

90. **The commonest neoplasm in an adult is :**
    A. Sarcoma   B. Papilloma
    C. Teratoma   D. Carcinoma

91. **Glomus tumor is usually found around finger nails or:**
    A. Tongue   B. Eye
    C. Ears   D. Umbilicus

92. **The edge of a basal cell carcinoma is :**
    A. Sloping   B. Everted
    C. Undermined   D. None of the above

93. **Treatment of Desmoid tumor is :**
    A. Surgery   B. Radiotherapy
    C. Radio + chemothrapy   D. Conservative treatment

94. **Which is not a tumor marker :**
    A. Beta-2 macroglobulin B. CEA
    C. Alpha fetoprotein   D. HCG

Ans.	83. C	84. C	85. D	86. D	87. A	88. B
	89. A	90. A	91. C	92. D	93. A	94. A

95. Match list 1 with 2 and select the correct answer using the codes given below the lists :

List 1
(Tumour markers)
I. Calcitonin
II. Alphafoetoprotein carcinoma thyroid
III. Carcinoembryonic antigen
IV. Alkaline phosphatase

List 2
(Diseases)
(i) Secondaries liver
(ii) Medullary
(iii) Malignant teratoma of yolk sac
(iv) Seminoma
(v) Carcinoma colon

A. I (i)   II (ii)   III (iii)   IV (iv)
B. I (ii)   II (iii)   III (v)   IV (i)
C. I (i)   II (iii)   III (iv)   IV (ii)
D. I (ii)   II (i)   III (v)   IV (iv)

96. A 32-year old mother of three children had noticed a dark discolouration under her right thumb nail for the past six months. The nail finally came off and was replaced by a draining ulcerated area with enlarged nodes appearing in the axilla. The most likely diagnosis is :
A. Melanoma   B. Phalangeal osteomyelitis
C. Sublingual haematoma   D. Glomus tumour

97. Not a premalignant ulcer :
A. Bazin's ulcer
B. Paget's disease of nipple
C. Marjolin's ulcer
D. Lupus vulgaris

98. Following are signs of internal malignancy except :
A. Tuberous sclerosis   B. Acanthosis nigricans
C. Dermatomyositis   D. All of the above

99. Sq. cell carcinoma is associated with :
A. Bowen's disease   B. Seborrhoeic keratosis
C. Lichen planus   D. Pemphigus vulgaris

100. The following organs have the lining of stratified squamous epithelium except :
A. Ureter   B. Pharynx
C. Vagina   D. Oesophagus

101. Most common site for lipoma to become malignant is :
A. Neck   B. Retroperitoneum
C. Legs   D. Viscera

Ans.   95. D   96. A   97. A   98. A   99. A   100. A
       101. B

102. **Which of the following neurofibroma is potentially threatening :**
  A. Multiple neurofibromatosis
  B. Acoustic neuroma
  C. Plexiform neurofibromatosis
  D. Generalised neurofibroma

103. **Evidence of early malignant change in a pigmented mole is :**
  A. Itching
  B. Rapid increase in size
  C. Satellite nodules
  D. All of the above

104. **Which of the following is not a feature of Marjolin's ulcer ?**
  A. Slow growth
  B. Found on previous scar
  C. Early metastatis
  D. Painless

105. **Glomus tumor is found in :**
  A. Adrenal gland
  B. Finger nails
  C. Liver
  D. Pituitary

106. **Carcinoma not metastasing to brain is of :**
  A. Nasopharynx
  B. Breast
  C. Lungs
  D. Liver

107. **True about chemodectoma is all except :**
  A. Lingual nerve palsy is often seen
  B. Origin from carotid
  C. Distant metastasis is rare
  D. Radioresistant

108. **Generalized lymphadenopathy is seen in following except :**
  A. CLL
  B. CML
  C. Hodgkin's lymphoma
  D. Non Hodgkin's lymphoma

109. **In Hodgkin's lymphoma, most commonly affected lymph nodes are :**
  A. Axillary
  B. Cervical
  C. Mediastinal
  D. Abdominal

110. **Which of the followng metastasises to lymph nodes :**
  A. Histiocytoma
  B. Angiosarcoma
  C. Fibrosarcoma
  D. Cavernous haemangioma

111. **CEA is increased in all except:**
  A. Lung Ca
  B. Melanoma
  C. Pancreatic Ca
  D. Colorectal Ca

112. **Most common site of malignant melanoma in males is :**
  A. Trunk
  B. Lower limb
  C. Toe
  D. Back

Ans.	102. B	103. D	104. C	105. B	106. A	107. A
	108. B	109. B	110. B	111. B	112. A	

113. **All are true about malignant melanoma except :**
A. Spontaneous regression
B. More in males
C. More common in albinism
D. Hentige maligna is least malignant

114. **Sentinel lymph node biopsy in an important part of the management of which of the following conditions :**
A. Cacinoma prostat   B. Carcinoma breast
C. Carcinoma lung   D. Carcinoma nosopharynx

115. **Tumor marker for endodermal sinus tumor is :**
A. CEA
B. AFP
C. Beta-HCG
D. Placental alkaline phophatase

116. **Match list I (disease conditions) and list II (tumor markers) and select the correct answer using the codes given below the list :**

List I		List II
A. Cancer breast	1.	CEA
B. Teratoma testis	2.	HER-2
C. Cancer colon	3.	HCG
D. Medullary thyroid cancer	4.	Calcification

Codes :
A. A2, B:3, C:1, D:4   B. A:4, B:1, C:3, D:2
C. A:2, B:1, C:3, D:4   D. A:4, B:3, C:1, D:2

117. **The following, except one are considered as cutaneous markers of internal malignancy:**
A. Acanthosis nigricans
B. Diffuse hyperpigmentation of the skin
C. Blue Iunule
D. Dermatomyositis in adults

118. **Least malignant potential is of :**
A. Sq. cell carcinoma   B. Basal cell carcinoma
C. Malignant malanoma   D. Epithelioma

119. **Which cutaneous malignancy does not metastasize to lymphatics :**
A. Basal cell carcinoma   B. Squamous cell carcinoma
C. Melanoma   D. Kaposi Sarcoma

120. **Margins of squamous cell carcinoma are :**
A. Inverted   B. Everted
C. Rolled   D. Undermined

Ans.	113. B	114. B	115. B	116. A	117. C	118. D
	119. A	120. B				

121. **True about rodent ulcer except :**
    A. Blood spread common
    B. Local invasion
    C. Healing and then recurrence
    D. Response to radiotherapy

122. **Internal malignancy is/are frequently associated with :**
    A. Erythema gyrum ripens
    B. Erythema chronicum migrans
    C. Erythema annular centrifugum
    D. All of the above

123. **Which of the following is of non-infective etiology :**
    A. Dermatitis herpetiformis   B. Erythrasma
    C. Ecthyma   D. Erysepeloid

124. **Following are precancerous dermatoses except :**
    A. Erythroplasia of Queyrat   B. Xeroderma pigmentosum
    C. Pigmented naevi   D. Senile lentigenes

125. **True about malignant melanoma true are except :**
    A. Acral lentigous is malignant
    B. Verticle thickness indicates prognosis
    C. Actinic keratosis is predisposing
    D. Spontaneous regression occurs

126. **Kaposi sarcoma, true is following except :**
    A. Rarely invasive
    B. Cutaneous vascular disease
    C. Koebner phenomenon seen
    D. Lymphnode involvement implies metastasis and poor prognosis

127. **The following malignancies can lead to erythroderma :**
    A. Carcinoma breast
    B. Bronchogenic carcinoma
    C. Hodgkin's disease
    D. Mycosis fungoides

128. **The most common type of carcinoma cutis in men originates from the :**
    A. Esophagus   B. Conjuctivae
    C. Larynx   D. Lung

129. **The most common type of carcinoma cutis in women originates from**   **the :**
    A. Esophagus   B. Larynx
    C. Lung   D. Breast

Ans.	121. A	122. A	123. A	124. D	125. C	126. D
	127. A	128. D	129. D			

130. Carcinoma cutis as the first sign of an internal cancer is most likely to occur with cancer of the :
    A. Breast, oral cavity, and stomach
    B. Breast, lung, and colon
    C. Lung, ovary, and kidney
    D. Breast, stomach, and lung

131. Preoperative topical application of which of the following may aid in visualization of tumor margins?
    A. Psoralen   B. Gentian violet
    C. 5-Fluorouracil   D. Potassium permanganate

132. Which histologic feature favors a diagnosis of extra-mammary over mammary Paget's disease?
    A. Signet ring cells
    B. Melanin within large atypical cells
    C. Multinucleated giant cells
    D. CEA positivity

133. The most common location for trichoepithelioma is the :
    A. Neck   B. Scalp
    C. Face   D. Back

134. Patients with Bloom's syndrome have an increased risk of which of the following malignancies except :
    A. Leukemia   B. Lymphoma
    C. Renal cell carcinoma   D. Gastrointestinal carcinoma

Ans.   130. C   131. C   132. A   133. C   — 134. C

CARDIOVASCULAR SYSTEM

1. **Cardiac myxoma commonly arises from :**
   A. Left Ventricle   B. Left Atrium
   C. Right Ventricle   D. Right Atrium

2. **The most common tumour of the heart is :**
   A. Myxoma   B. Angioma
   C. Mesothelioma   D. Rhabdomyoma

3. **The common primary tumor of heart :**
   A. Rhabdomyoma   B. Fibroma
   C. Myxoma   D. Lipoma

4. **Commonest tumor to metastasize to heart :**
   A. Malignant melanoma   B. Leomyosarcoma
   C. Osteogenic Ca   D. Carcinoid

5. **Commonest benign and malignant primary tumors of veins are :**
   A. Leiomyoma; Leiomyosarcoma
   B. Haemangiomas
   C. Chemodectoma
   D. Hydroma

6. **Which of the following histological types of lung cancer is associated with the myasthenic (Eaton-Lambert) syndrome?**
   A. Adenocarcinoma   B. Epidermoid carcinoma
   C. Large cell carcinoma   D. Small cell carcinoma

7. **The most favourable pulmonary metastatic lesions include all except :**
   A. Breast   B. Kidney
   C. Testis   D. Uterus
   E. Melanoma

8. **Which of the following is the commonest cause of calcified pulmonary metastasis :**
   A. Adenocarcinoma kidney   B. Squamous cell carcinoma
   C. Seminoma   D. Carcinoma thyroid

9. **Which of the following is the commonest tumor of anterior mediastinum :**
   A. Thymoma   B. Neurofibroma
   C. Ectopic thyroid   D. Lymphoma

Ans.	1. B	2. A	3. C	4. A	5. B	6. D
	7. E	8. D	9. A			

10. In a patient of mesothelioma, one often finds :
   A. Hypoglycaemia
   B. An association with asbestosis
   C. Haemorrhagic pleural effusion
   D. Clubbing of fingers
   E. All of the above

11. Ganglioneuroma is most common in :
   A. Ant. mediastinum
   B. Middle mediastinum
   C. Post. mediastinum
   D. Retroperitoneum region

12. Bronchogenic carcinoma commonly metastatise to which endocrine organ :
   A. Ovaries   B. Testes
   C. Thyroid   D. Adrenals

13. All of the following are anterior mediastinal tumours except :
   A. Thymoma   B. Teratoma
   C. Neurofibroma   D. Retrosternal goitre

14. A coin shaped lesion in apical lobes with erosion of ribs and thoracic vertebra is :
   A. Coarctation of aorta   B. Pancoast tumour
   C. Bronchiectesis   D. Any of the above

15. The most common mediastinal tumour is :
   A. Neurogenic tumour   B. Bronchogenic carcinoma
   C. Plasma cell myelomas D. Pericardial cysts

16. Myxoma is most common in :
   A. Left atrium   B. Right atrium
   C. Left ventricle D. Right ventricle

17. Ca lung mainly metastasize to :
   A. Liver   B. Brain
   C. Bone   D. Skin

18. Lung carcinoma and nonsmoking indicates :
   A. Multifactorial etiology   B.Unifactorial etiology
   C. Unpredictable associatio D.   No association

19. Pancoast tumor produces :
   A. Marked Erythema   B. Horner's syndrome
   C. Monoplegia   D. Hemiparesis

20. The most common type of bronchogenic carcinoma is :
   A. Epidermoid   B. Anaplastic
   C. Alveolar   D. Bronchiolar

Ans.	10. E	11. D	12. D	13. C	14. B	15. B
	16. A	17. A	18. A	19. B	20. A	

21. **All are true with bronchial adenoma except :**
   A. Uncommon benign tumours of the bronchus
   B. 10% of them are malignant
   C. 80% of them arise from a major bronchus
   D. They produce localized emphysema

22. **Which of the following often metastasizes to oppste lung?**
   A. Epidermoid carcinoma B. Alveolar cell carcinoma
   C. Adenocarcinoma D. Carcinoid

23. **The Chemotherapy is most useful for :**
   A. Squamous cell carcinoma
   B. Oat cell carcinoma
   C. Adenocarcinoma
   D. Neuroblastoma

24. **Cavity formation in bronchogenic carcinoma occurs in :**
   A. Oat cell carcinoma
   B. Squamous cell carinoma
   C. Adenocarcinoma
   D. Bronchoalveolar carcinoma

25. **Bronchogenic carcinoma which produce paraneo-plastic syndrome :**
   A. Squamous cell carcinoma B. Oat cell carcinoma
   C. Adenocarcinoma D. Large cell carcinoma

26. **Commonest tumor to metastasise to heart is :**
   A. Malignant melanoma B. Bronchogenic carcinoma
   C. Ca breast D. Leomysarcoma

27. **Common cause of SVC obstruction is :**
   A. Thrombosis B. Extrinsic compression
   C. Congenital web D. Neoplastic encroachment

28. **Least likely cause of lung secondaries is :**
   A. Ca breast B. Ca testis
   C. Ca ovary D. Ca prostate

29. **The commonest tumor associated with acquired pure red cell aplasia is :**
   A. Bronchogenic carcinoma B. Hepatic carcinoma
   C. Hodgkin's lymphoma D. Thymoma

30. **Investigation of choice in a solitary pulmonary nodule is :**
   A. High resolution CT scan
   B. MRI
   C. Contrast enhanced CT scan
   D. Image guided FNAC

Ans.	21. A	22. C	23. B	24. B	25. B	26. A
	27. D	28. D	29. D	30. A		

31. **True adenocarcinoma of esophagus is most likely to be due to :**
    A. Achalasia
    B. Barret's esophagus
    C. Patterson Brown syndrome
    D. Scleroderma

32. **The following are true about bronchogenic carcinoma except :**
    A. It is the commonest malignant tumour in men
    B. One-Lung-Anaesthesia has improved results of surgery
    C. Most lung cancers are unresectable at presentation
    D. Small cell carcinoma carries better survival rate

33. **'Popcorn' calcification in a lung nodule is pathognomic of :**
    A. Hamartomas   B. Histoplasmosis
    C. Tuberculosis   D. Benign nodule

34. **A 60 year old male was diagnosed as carcinoma right lung. On CECT chest there was a tumor of 5´5 cm in upper lobe and another 2´2 cms size tumor nodule in middle lobe. The primary modality of treatment is?**
    A. Radiotherapy   B. Chemotherapy
    C. Surgery   D. Supportive treatment

35. **Poorest prognosis in lung cancer is associated with :**
    A. Small cell carcinoma
    B. Squamous cell carcinoma
    C. Squamous cell carcinoma
    D. Adenosquamous carcinoma

Ans.	31. B	32. D	33. A	34. C	35. A

RESPIRATORY SYSTEM

1. **Malignant tumur of the lung may be of any of the following types except :**
    A. Squamous cell carcinoma
    B. Anaplastic carcinoma
    C. Clear cell carcinoma
    D. Adenocarcinoma
    E. Epidermoid carcinoma

2. **Cigarette smoking predisposes to which of the following lung cancer :**
    A. Adenocarcinoma   B. Squamous cell carcinoma
    C. Oat cell carcinoma   D. b + c
    E. All of the above

3. **Bronchogenic carcinoma may spread to the following except :**
    A. Liver   B. Kidneys
    C. Adrenal   D. Gall Bladder

4. **Which of the following is not a histological type of carcinoma lung :**
    A. Small cell   B. Oat cell
    C. Squamous cell D. Transitional type

5. **Commonest type of bronchogenic carcinoma is :**
    A. Adenocarcinoma
    B. Oat cell carcinoma
    C. Squamous cell carcinoma
    D. Large cell carcinoma

6. **Mesothelioma of pleura is commonly associated with :**
    A. Asbestosis   B. Anthracosis
    C. Silicosis   D. Siderosis

7. **Which is associated with Ca Lung :**
    A. Chromium   B. Berrylium
    C. Asbestosis   D. Nickel

8. **The type of bronchogenic Ca with best prognosis is :**
    A. Oat cell   B. Small cell
    C. Large cell   D. Squamous cell carcinoma

Ans.	1. C	2. D	3. D	4. D	5. A	6. A
	7. C	8. D				

9. **Paramalignant effusion is seen in :**
   A. Hypoproteinemia
   B. Lymphatic block
   C. Malignancy related cachexia
   D. Bronchogenic carcinoma

10. **The lung carcinoma most common in non smokers is :**
   A. Sq. cell   B. Large cell
   C. Adenocarcinoma   D. Small cell

11. **A man has Ca lung with nephrotic syndrome of type :**
   A. Mesangial type
   B. Minimal type
   C. Membranous type
   D. Mesangio proliferative type

12. **All of the following paraneoplastic syndromes are seen in Bronchogenic carcinoma except :**
   A. Myasesthenia gravis
   B. Hypocalcemia
   C. Hyperparathyroidism
   D. Hypertrophic pulmonary osteoarthropathy

13. **The type of carcinoma arising from the scars of the lung :**
   A. Squamous cell carcinoma
   B. Oat cell carcinoma
   C. Adenocarcinoma
   D. Undifferentiated carcinoma

14. **Scar in lung tissue develops into :**
   A. Adenocarcinoma
   B. Oat cell Carcinoma
   C. Squamous cell Carcinoma
   D. Columnar cell carcinoma

15. **On an autopsy specimen of lung tissue, stratified squamous epithelium was noted in the bronchi. Which among the following would best describe its presence**
   A. Metaplasia   B. Hyperplasia
   C. Dysplasia   D. Hyperplasia

16. **The most common underlying scar for scar carcinoma in lungs is:**
   A. Infaract   B. Granuloma
   C. Tuberculoma   D. Fibrotic scar.

17. **Typical carcinoid in lung presents as :**
   A. Lobar collapse   B. Obstructive pneumonitis
   C. Hilar mass   D. Any of the above.

Ans.	9. B	10. C	11. C	12. B	13. C	14. A
	15. A	16. A	17. D			

18. Cavitating pulmonary metastases are usually from:
    A. Testes   B. Colon
    C. Kidneys   D. Cervix

19. Primary lung cancer is unlikely if a solitary pulmonary nodule:
    A. Has well-defined margins
    B. Has spiculated margins
    C. Contains pleural tag
    D. There is no growth for at least 2 years.

20. Pancoast tumour is more commonly seen in type:
    A. Squamous   B. Columnar
    C. Adeno   D. Pseudostratified

21. The cause of single coin shadow in the lung with calcification in the center is :
    A. Epidermoid carcinoma B. Adeno carcinoma
    C. Melanoma   D. Oat cell tumour

22. The most common malignant tumour of the lung in smokers is:
    A. Fibrosarcoma   B. Adenocarcinoma
    C. Leiomyosarcoma   D. Squamous cell carcinoma

23. Malignant thymoma most commonly spreads to :
    A. Brain   B. Spine
    C. Pleura   D. Liver

24. All are superior mediastinal tumors except:
    A. Thymoma
    B. Pleurodermoid cyst
    C. Branchial cyst
    D. Extra-adrenal phaeochromocytoma

25. Diagnostic sign in carcinoma lung in Chest X-ray is :
    A. Rib erosion
    B. Central destruction within the lesion
    C. Flattening of diaphragm
    D. Elevation of diaphragm

26. The characteristic X-ray feature of pancoast tumour is :
    A. Coin shadow
    B. Apical consolidation
    C. Apical mass lesion with erosion of neck of 1 & 2 ribs
    D. Hilar mass

27. Incidence of pulmonary metastasis is maximum with:
    A. Choriocarcinoma   B. Wilm's tumor
    C. Ewing's tumor   D. Seminoma

Ans.	18. D	19. D	20. A	21. A	22. D	23. C
	24. C	25. A	26. C	27. A		

28. **Commonest malignant tumour of chest wall in children is:**
   A. Neuroblastoma
   B. Ewing sarcoma
   C. Rhabdomiosarcoma
   D. Lymphosarcoma
29. **Cavitatory lesions in lung are seen in following except :**
   A. Malignant melanoma
   B. Ca cervix
   C. Renal cell carcinoma
   D. Osteosarcoma

Ans. 28. B   29. D

GASTROINTESTINAL SYSTEM

1. **The commonest benign solid epithelial tumor of liver is :**
   A. Hamartoma
   B. Adenoma
   C. Papilloma
   D. Cystadenoma
   E. Bile duct adenanas

2. **Commonest histological type of anal carcinoma is :**
   A. Adenocarcinoma
   B. Squamous cell
   C. Transitional cell carcinoma
   D. Columnar

3. **Commonest variety of carcinoma stomach is :**
   A. Squamous carcinoma
   B. Adenocarcinoma
   C. Colloid carcinoma
   D. None

4. **Mesenchymal benign tumours of the stomach include the following except :**
   A. Leiomyoma
   B. Adenoma
   C. Fibroma
   D. Lipoma
   E. Hemangioma

5. **Adenomyomas of gall bladder are always located in :**
   A. Fundus
   B. Neck
   C. Hartman's pouch
   D. Bile duct

6. **Commonest carcinoma of bile duct is :**
   A. Sclerosing adenocarcinoma
   B. Papillary adenocarcinoma
   C. Keratinizing sq. cell carcinomas
   D. Adenomatous polyp

7. **All the following are produced by carcinoids except :**
   A. Serotonin
   B. 5 hydroxytryptophan
   C. Bradykinin
   D. Histamine

8. **Of the following colonic polyps, which has least malignant potential ?**
   A. Juvenile polyps
   B. Gardner's syndrome
   C. Familial polyposis
   D. Turcot's syndrome

9. **The polyps in colon more prone for malignancy :**
   A. Villous
   B. Lobular
   C. Both are equally prone
   D. None of the above

Ans.	1. A	2. B	3. B	4. B	5. A	6. A
	7. B	8. A	9. A			

10. **Pancreatic carcinoma is least common in :**
    A. Tail   B. Body
    C. Head   D. Diffused

11. **Cholangio-carcinoma :**
    A. Undifferentiated carcinoma usually
    B. Evokes abundant fibroblastic proliferation
    C. Bile present within tumour cells
    D. All of the above

12. **Villous adenomas are most frequently seen in :**
    A. caecum   B. Ascending colon
    C. Transverse colon   D. Rectum

13. **Most malignant gastric tumour is :**
    A. Lymphoma
    B. Adenocarcinoma
    C. Leiomyosarcoma
    D. Squamous cell carcinoma
    E. Columnar cell carcinoma

14. **Hamartomatous polypi in colon are seen in :**
    A. Peutz-Jeghers syndrome
    B. Canada-Chronkhite syndrome
    C. Gardner's syndrome
    D. Turcot's syndrome

15. **Hepatic adenomas are associated with :**
    A. Cirrhosis   B. Vinyl chloride
    C. Oral contraceptives   D. Aflatoxins

16. **Which of the following statements is False regarding hepatoma :**
    A. It is more common in males
    B. Cirrhosis of liver is a predisposing factor
    C. They commonly metastasize
    D. Alkaline phosphatase is markedly elevated

17. **The following statement is correct about 'CEA' :**
    A. Used to screen patients with HCC
    B. Used as a tumour marker for colonic carcinoma and to follow up patient post opertively after resolution of tumor
    C. Used to determine prognosis in patients with Hodgkins d/s
    D. None

18. **The most definite indication of malignant transfor-mation of a benign polyp of colon is :**
    A. Infilteration of fibrous core
    B. Infilteration of base of polyp
    C. Ulceration at the tip of polyp
    D. Lymphatic permeation

Ans.	10. A	11. B	12. D	13. B	14. A	15. C
	16. C	17. B	18. A			

19.   **Most common benign tumour to stomach is :**
      A. Lipoma   B. Fibroma
      C. Leiomyoma   D. Rhabdomyomas

20.   **Most common site of carcinoid with liver metastasis :**
      A. Appendix   B. Ileum
      C. Ovary   D. Jejunum

21.   **Commonest oral cancer is :**
      A. Squanous cell type   B. Adeno carcinoma
      C. Transitional cell type D. Columnar cell carcinoma

22.   **The commonest secondary in spleen is :**
      A. Gall bladder adenocarcinoma
      B. Carcinoma kidney
      C. Melanoma
      D. Carcinoma Prostate

23.   **Multiple gastric ulcers and hypertrophied mucosa   are seen in :**
      A. Zollinger Ellison syndrome
      B. Pyloric stenosis
      C. Pernicious anaemia
      D. Malignant ulcer

24.   **Which of the following is most often associated with carcinoma stomach :**
      A. Pernicious anemia   B. Acute gastritis
      C. Chronic gastritis   D. Duodenal ulcer

25.   **A premalignant condition for carcinoma liver is :**
      A. Hepatitis B virus   B. Schistosomiasis
      C. Smoking   D. Coxsackie virus

26.   **Primary tumors are rare in :**
      A. Oesophagus   B. Stomach
      C. Small bowel   D. Large bowel

27.   **An incidental finding at an autopsy was a round, well-circumscribed mass in the liver. It was composed of cords liver cells with sinusoids and bile ducts in a disorderly pattern that represented essentially a focal overgrowth of normal liver tissue. The best classification for this mass would be :**
      A. Carcinoma   B. Choristoma
      C. Hamartoma   D. Teratoma

28.   **Hour glass deformity is seen in :**
      A. Carcinoma stomach   B. Peptic ulcer
      C. Duodenal atresia   D. Ch. pyloric stenosis
      E. All of the above

Ans.	19. C	20. B	21. A	22. C	23. A	24. A
	25. A	26. C	27. C	28. B		

29. Carcinoma stomach with best prognosis is :
    A. Suferficial spreading B. Ulcerative
    C. Polypoidal fungating D. Linitus plastica
30. The most malignant tumor of appendix is :
    A. Argentaffinoma   B. Adenocarcinoma
    C. a+b   D. None of the above
31. The most common tumour of appendix is :
    A. Lymphoma   B. Adenocarcinoma
    C. Fibrosarcoma   D. Argentaffinoma
32. The colon is thickened; the mucosa presents cobblestone' appearance with linear ulcers. There are giant cells in the regional lymphnodes. The most likely disease is :
    A. Carcinoma of colon   B. Amoebic colitis
    C. Ulcerative colitis   D. Crohn's disease
33. Malignant potential of colonic polyp is suggested by :
    A. Juvenile polyp
    B. Tubular polyp
    C. A larger tubulovillous component
    D. Hamartomatrus polyp
34. Which of the following pancreatic tumor is most commonly seen in MEN type I :
    A. Gastrinoma   B. Glucagonoma
    C. Insulinoma   D. Somatostatinom
35. Most common malignancy of hepatic nodule :
    A. Hemangioma   B. Hepatic adenoma
    C. Cholangio adenoma   D. Hepatocarcinoma
36. Carcinoid syndrome is not seen in :
    A. Oesophagus   B. Duodenum
    C. Stomach   D. Intestine
37. Hepatocellular carcinoma is characterized by all except :
    A. Jaundice   B. Hepatomegaly
    C. ↑ Alk. phosphatase   D. ↓ alpha fetoprotei
38. Carcinoma tongue is :
    A. Adenocarcinoma
    B. Squamous cell carcinoma
    C. Stratified squamous cell carcinoma
    D. None of the above
39. Most common site for extra nodal lymphoma is :
    A. Liver   B. Stomach
    C. Small bowel   D. Large bowel

Ans.	29. A	30. B	31. D	32. D	33. B	34. A
	35. A	36. A	37. A	38. B	39. B	

40. **Perineurual infilteration in parotid tumors is seen in :**
    A. Adenolymphoma   B. Adenoid cystic
    C. Cylindrioma   D. Mixed paratod tumor
41. **Histology of lip carcinoma :**
    A. Adenolymphoma   B. Squamus cell carcinoma
    C. Mucoid cystic   D. Cylindroma
42. **The worst prognosis is associated with :**
    A. A fungating or polypoidal carcinoma of the stomach
    B. An ulcer cancer of the stomach
    C. A superficial spreading cancer of the stomach
    D. Linitis plastica of the stomach
43. **The most common site of carcinoma of the colon is :**
    A. Cecum   B. Ascending colon
    C. Transverse colon   D. Rectosigmoid
44. **Leather bottle stomach is the result of :**
    A. Achlorhydria   B. Hypertrophic gastritis
    C. Ulcerative carcioma   D. Diffuse carcinoma
45. **Commonest malignancy of the small intestine is :**
    A. Adenocarcinoma   B. Lymphoma
    C. Carcinoid   D. Leiomysosarcoma
46. **Which of the following is false regarding Argentaf- in tumours of the small intestine :**
    A. It is an epithelial tumour of small bowel
    B. It is usually single
    C. It can cause carcinoid syndrome when the liver is involved.
    D. All of the above are correct
47. **The most common malignant tumor involving the liver is :**
    A. Hepatoblastoma   B. Angiosarcoma
    C. Heaptocellular carcinoma   D.Mestastatic carcinoma
48. **The most common premalignant lesion in large intestine is :**
    A. Juvenile polyp   B. Villous adenoma
    C. Hyperplastic polyp   D. Peutz-Jegher's polyp
49. **The carcinoma of Pancreas usually originate in the :**
    A. Duct epithelium   B. Aberrant pancreas
    C. Stroma   D. Islets of Langerhans
50. **Most common site of leiomyoma is :**
    A. Stomach   B. Ileum
    C. Colon   D. Trauma
51. **Nesidioblastoma is a tumour of :**
    A. D-cells of pancreas   B. β-cells of pancreas
    C. α-cells of pancreas   D. Exocrine pancreas

Ans.	40. B	41. B	42. D	43. D	44. D	45. A
	46. B	47. D	48. B	49. A	50. A	51. B

52. **Which of the following about 'Promoters' in carcinogenesis is true ?**
   A. Promoters of tumor suppression
   B. A carcinogenic agent by itself
   C. Enhances the rapidity of onset/yield of the tumor
   D. Promotor of benign tumors
   E. Promotor of the formation of a second tumor

53. **The characteristic features of hepatoblastoma include all the following except :**
   A. Small fusiform embryonal type cells
   B. Large foetal cells with more cytoplasm
   C. Synthesis of Alpha Foeto Protein by the tumor cells
   D. Secretion of Carcino Embryonic Antigen
   E. Recurrence of extramedullary haemopoiesis

54. **All of the following are true regarding fibrolamellar cancer of the liver except :**
   A. More in women
   B. Better prognosis than HCC
   C. Increase AFP
   D. All of the above

55. **There is no predisposition for carcinom change in :**
   A. Ulcerative colitis   B. Amoebic colitis
   C. Familial polyposis   D. Sclerosing colangitis

56. **All are premalignant conditions of oesophagus except :**
   A. Varices   B. Barrett's ocsophagus
   C. Achalasia cardia   D. Plummer vinson syndrome

57. **Most common cause of benign strictures in oesophagus is :**
   A. Achalasia cardia
   B. Foreign body in oesophagus
   C. Strictures due to caustics & alkalies
   D. Congenital

58. **True about carcinoma esophagus is :**
   A. Most common site lower end
   B. Both adeno and squamous cell carcinoma occur
   C. Commonest histology adenocarcinoma
   D. More common in females

59. **Which is true regarding Barret's oesophagus :**
   A. Squamous metaplasia of lower esophagus
   B. Seen mainly in females
   C. Premalignant
   D. Responds to conservative management

Ans.	52. C	53. D	54. C	55. B	56. A	57. C
	58. B	59. C				

60. True about Ca Esophagus :
A. Multicentric
B. Commonest in upper one third
C. Submucosal spread not common
D. Colon is used for reconstruction

61. Adenocarcinoma oesophagus, following is true :
A. Ba emulsion is used for diagnosis
B. Occurs mostly in lower 1/3
C. Upper 1/3 commonly involved
D. Radiotherapy useful

62. Commonest cause of death in Ca oesophagus anastomosis by Ivor Lewis method is :
A. Anastomatic leak
B. Anastomatic necrosis
C. Pulm. atelectasis
D. Myocarditis

63. True about Ca Esophagus :
A. Mostly stenotic
B. Histology of tumour indicates prognosis
C. Perirectal involvement is treated by local resection
D. Spread to adjacent tissue affects the final prognosis after surgery

64. Esophageal carcinoma most commonly occurs at :
A. Upper third   B. Middle third
C. Lower third   D. Post cricoid region

65. Commonest benign tumour of the esophagus is :
A. Leiomyoma   B. Papilloma
C. Adenoma   D. Hemangioma

66. The commonest type of presentation of carcinoma oesophagus is :
A. Stricturous growth   B. Cauliflower growth
C. Infilterating growth   D. Polypoid growth

67. Which one of the following statements about neoplasia in the oesophagus is correct ?
A. Benign tumours are more frequent than carcinomas
B. Metastatic spread is not an important feature of carcinoma of the oesophagus
C. Massive haematemesis is a feature of oesophageal carcinoma
D. Adenocarcinomas of the proximal stomach can invade the lower end of the oesophagus and cause Dysphagia

Ans.	60. D	61. B	62. A	63. B	64. B	65. A
	66. D	67. D				

68. A 32-year old woman had been troubled by progressive dysphagia for several years with the necessity to drink water to force food down. There had been no weight loss or loss of appetite but sometimes there was voluminous regurgitation after meals. Recently, there have been several bouts of pneumonia. The most likely diagnosis is :
    A. Oesophageal hiatal hernia
    B. Achalasia cardia
    C. Carcinoma of oesophagus
    D. Stricuture of oesophagus

69. Most common site for squamous ca esophagus :
    A. Upper third
    B. Mid third
    C. Lower third
    D. Cricoesophageal junction

70. True adenocarcinoma of esophagus is most likely to be due to :
    A. Achalasi
    B. Barret's esophagus
    C. Patterson Brown syndrome
    D. Scleroderma

71. Which of the following is diagnostic of carcinoma stomach ?

    A. Bleeding per rectum
    B. Plain X-ray abdomen
    C. Barium meal
    D. Gastroscopy

72. Carcinoma stomach at the pyloric end in a manageable condition should be managed by :
    A. Upper radical partial gastrectomy
    B. Lower radical partial gastrectomy
    C. Gastro-jejunostomy
    D. Radiotherapy

73. Presenting symptom of carcinoma stomach is :
    A. Weight loss
    B. Perforation
    C. Bleeding
    D. Obstruction

74. All of the following are true of leimyosarcoma of the stomach except :
    A. Histological diagnosisis easily obtained by endoscopic biopsy
    B. They are asymptomatic until they become very large
    C. They commonly present with pain and occult or massive haemorrhage
    D. They arise more commonly from the proximal stomach

75. Krukenberg tumour of ovary arises from :
    A. Breast
    B. Stomach
    C. Liver
    D. Rectum

Ans.	68. B	69. B	70. B	71. D	72. B	73. A
	74. A	75. B				

76. **Rx of gastric adenocarcinoma is :**
A. Surgery with Chemotherpay
B. Chemotherapy
C. Radiotherapy/Chemotherapy
D. Preoperative RT with surgery

77. **Consider the following statements :**
In carcinoma of the stomach
1. A fixed abdominal lump indicates inoperability
2. Radiotherapy offers a good chance of cure
3. In advanced disease, paliative resection is better than palliative bypass operation
A. 1,2 and 3 are correct   B.   1 and 2 are correct
C. 2 and 3 are correct   D.   1 and 3 are correct

78. **Hour glass deformity of the stomach is seen in :**
A. Gastric ulcer   B.   Gastric carcinoma
C. Gastric lymphoma   D.   Corrosive strictures

79. **The most common benign tumor of the Stomach is :**
A. Leiomyoma   B.   Adenoma
C. Hamartoma   D.   Lipoma

80. **Most common site of Carcinoma stomach is :**
A. Fundus   B.   Pylorus
C. Antrum   D.   Cardia

81. **Erosive gastritis can predispose to Carcinoma stomach at following sites except :**
A. Lesser curvature   B.   Antrum
C. Body   D.   Fundus

82. **Treatment of Zollinger Ellison syndrome is :**
A. Total gastrectomy   B.   Partial gastrectomy
C. Excision of tumor alone   D.H2 receptor antagonist

83. **Which of the following is not true about uncomplicated benign gastric ulcers ?**
A. Commonly recur after medical treatment
B. Should receive surgical treatment it healing has not occurred after 4 to 6 weeks of medical treatment
C. Occur most commonly on the greater curvature
D. Should initially be treated medically

84. **Which of the following is not related clinically or pathologically to carcinoma of the stomach ?**
A. Blood group O   B.   Troisier's sign
C. Linitis plastica   D.   Krukenberg tumours

Ans.	76. A	77. D	78. A	79. A	80. B	81. D
	82.	83. C	84. A			

85. The prognosis following resection of carcinoma of the stomach is determined by :
    A. The extent of stomach removed
    B. The margin of apparently healthy stomach removed above the growth
    C. A short clinical history
    D. The histology of the growth

86. The following are the common presentations of adenomatous polyp in stomach except :
    A. Bleeding   B. Abdominal pain
    C. Vomiting (bile stained) D. Achlorhydria

87. The following the premalignant potential of adenomatous polypus of stomach :
    A. Multiple
    B. Associated pernicious anaemia
    C. Recurrence
    D. All of the above

88. The following indicate the premalignant potential of adenomatous polypus of stomach :
    A. Multiple
    B. Associated Pernicious anaemia
    C. Recurrence
    D. All of the above

89. Adequate margins of resection are essential for gastrectomy for carcinoma. With positive margins, the 5-year survival rate is less than 15. Ideal margins both proximal and distal are at least :
    A. 4 cm   B. 6 cm
    C. 8 cm   D. 10 cm
    E. 12 cm

90. Carcinoma stomach with good prognosis is :
    A. Superficial spreading B. Ulcerative
    C. Fungating type   D. Linitus plastica

91. Barium meal picture of carcinoma stomach shows following :
    A. Filling defect
    B. Loss of rugosity
    C. Small capacity of stomach
    D. Delayed emptying barium
    E. All of the above

92. All of the following predispose to gastric carcinoma except :
    A. Achlorhydia   B. 'O' blood group
    C. Pernicious anaemia   D. Post gastrectomy

Ans.	85. D	86. C	87. D	88. D	89. B	90. A
	91. E	92. B				

93. Which of the following signs are present in an advanced case of carcinoma of stomach ?
    1. Trousseau's sign
    2. Troisier's sign
    3. Depostis in the pouch of Douglas
    4. Murphy's sign
    Select the correct answer :
    A. 1 and 4   B. 1 and 2
    C. 1,2 and 3   D. 2,3 and 4

94. **Commonest site of Leimyoma in GIT is :**
    A. Stomach   B. Ileum
    C. Jejunum   D. Rectum

95. **Troiser's sign is seen in all except :**
    A. Ca stomach   B. Seminoma
    C. Medulloblastoma   D. Ca Pancreas

96. **Consider the following types of growths :**
    1. Pyloric growth
    2. Carcinoma of body of stomach
    3. Growth at cardia
    The correct sequence in Descending order of the degree of accuracy of barium meal examination for the diagnosis of carcinoma stomach in respect of the given types of growths is :
    A. 2,1,3   B. 3,1,2
    C. 1,2,3   D. 1,3,2

97. **Early gastric carcinoma is :**
    A. Mucosa involved without lymph node involvement
    B. Mucosa involved irrespective of lymph node involvement
    C. Submucosa involved irrespective of lymph node involvement
    D. Submucosa involved without lymph node involvement

98. **Treatment of choice of a tumor 5 cm size present in prepyloric region of stomach is :**
    A. Entrectomy   B. Subtotal gastrectomy
    C. Total gastrectomy   D. Gastrojejunal anastomosis

99. **Gastric malignancy is predisposed with :**
    A. Duodenal ulce
    B. Gastric hyperplasia
    C. Intestinal metaplasia III
    D. Blood group O

Ans.	93. C	94. A	95. C	96. A	97. C	98. B
	99. C					

100. All the following indicates early gastric cancer except :
   A. Involvement of mucosa
   B. Involvement of mucosa and submucosa
   C. Involvement of mucosa, submucosa and muscularis
   D. Involvement of mucosa, submucosa and adjacent lymph nodes

101. Carcinoma pancreas is most common in :
   A. The body of pancreas
   B. The tail of pancreas
   C. The periampullary region of head
   D. The head proper
   E. Ampulla of Vater

102. 'Lead paint' appearance of stool in a jaundiced patient indicates :
   A. Carcinoma of the head proper of pancreas
   B. Carcinoma of the tail pancreas
   C. Carcinoma of periampullary region of pancreas
   D. Cholecystitis along with haemorrhage
   E. Jaundice with intoxication due to lead paints

103. Secondaries to liver can arise from the following sites except :
   A. Lungs   B. Kidney
   C. Stomach   D. Breast

104. The commonest pancratic tumour is :
   A. Ductal adenocarcinoma
   B. Cystadenoma
   C. Insulinoma
   D. Non islet cell tumour

105. Cholangiocarcinoma histological resembles :
   A. Sq. cell type   B. Colloid cell type
   C. Schirrhous type   D. Columnar cell type

106. Chemotherapeutic agent of choice in Ca. pancreas is :
   A. Mitomycin-C   B. 5-FU
   C. Adriamycin   D. Streptozocin

107. Which of the following is not a possible etiological factor in the case of hepatocellular carcinoma :
   A. Mycotoxin   B. Plant alkaloid
   C. Oral contraceptive D. Androgens
   E. Aspirin

108. Which of the following histological type of hepatocellular carcinoma carries the best   prognosis :
   A. Trabecular type   B. Pseudoglandular type
   C. Schirrhous type   D. Pleomorphic type
   E. Fibrolamellar type

Ans.	100. C	101. D	102. C	103. B	104. A	105. C
	106. D	107. E	108. E			

109. **Liver cell adenoma and focal nodular hyperplasia of liver have following similarities except :**
A. Occur primarily in women
B. Occur predominantly at older age group
C. Have relation with oral contraceptive intake
D. Both are composed of hepatocytes

110. **In insulinoma, following are seen except : Rajasthan 1998**
A. Hypoglycenoid
B. Loss of body weight
C. Cardiac arrythmias
D. Relieved with I/V glucose

111. **Hepatocellular carcinoma may be a complicaiton of following except :**
A. Pain last for several hours
B. Serum amylase levels corrlates with severity of attack
C. Common in alcoholics
D. Low serum calcium levels indicate good prognosis

112. **The commonest manifestation of carcinoma head of pancreas is :**
A. Palpable mass   B. Obstructive jaundice
C. Steatorrhoea   D. Pain

113. **Alpha foetoproteins in hepatoblastoma are seen in   about :**
A. One third cases   B. Two third cases
C. 90%   D. 100%

114. **Klatskin tumour is situated at :**
A. At ehe junction of Right & left hepatic duct   –
B. At the lower end of common hepatic duct
C. At the lower end of common bile duct
D. At porta hepatis

115. **Carcinoma of pancreas attains greatest size when it is located in :**
A. Head   B. Body and tail
C. Ampullary region   D. Ampulla of Vater

116. **The commonest tumour in liver is :**
A. Secondaries   B. Hepatoma
C. Haemangioma   •   D. None of the above

117. **Investigation of choice in Ca ampulla of vater is :**
A. Ba meal follow through
B. ERCP
C. Enzyme essay
D. Radionuclide pancreatic scan

Ans.	109. B	110. B	11. C	112. B	113. B	114. A
	115. B	116. A	117. D			

118. True about hepatocellular carcinoma is following except :
    A. Uncommon in Asians
    B. Aflatoxin
    C. Hepatitis B & C markers increased
    D. Fibrolamellar type has better prognosis
119. Cholangiocarcinoma is seen in following except :
    A. Sclerosing cholangitis B. Clonorchis sinensis
    C. Gall stones   D. Ulcerative colitis
120. Feature common to carcinoma pancreas, lungs, stomach is :
    A. Thrombophlebitis
    B. Migratory thrombophlebitis
    C. Ascites
    D. DIC
121. Commonest malignancy of spleen is :
    A. Lymphoma   B. Metaststic ca colon
    C. Metastastic ca kidney D. Splenic hemangioma
122. Which of the following regarding pancreatic carcinoma is false ?
    A. Most frequent symptoms are weight loss, pain and anorexia
    B. More than 75 percent of all cases are Adenocarcinomas of ductal cell origin
    C. The ratio of the Head & Neck tumors compared to body and tail is 1 : 2
    D. The prevalence of jaundice varies with the position in the pancreas where the tumour is situated
    E. At the time of presentation disease is beyond surgical resection in over 80 percent of cases
123. Most common malignant tumor of spleen is :
    A. Lymphoma   B. Haemangioma
    C. Adenocarcinoma   D. Sq. cell carcinoma
124. Pancreatic Ca is caused by :
    A. Fasciola   B. Clonorchis
    C. Paragonimus   D. Granulosus
125. All the following are true regarding fibrolamellar carcinoma of the liver except :
    A. AFP levels > 1000
    B. It occurs in younger individuals
    C. More common in females
    D. Better prognosis as compared to HCC
126. Insulinoma most commonly occurs in :
    A. Head of pancreas
    B. Body of pancreas

Ans.	118. A	119. C	120. B	121. A	122. E	123. A
	124. B	125. A	126. C			

C. Tail of pancreas
D. Equally distributed in head, body and tail

127. **In intestine, lipoma is commonest in :**
    A. Rectum   B. Sigmoid colon
    C. Calcum   D. Ileum

128. **Recognised features of the carcinoid syndrome include all of the following except :**
    A. Constipation
    B. Pellagra
    C. Precipitation of attacks by alcohol ingestion
    D. Wheezing

129. **Treatment of choice of umbilical adenoma (2.5 x 1.5 cm) in a new born is :**
    A. Occlusion with a coin
    B. Strapping
    C. Surgery
    D. Leave as such as regression occurs

130. **Tumours which have a tendency towards direct extension through tissue spaces include following, except :**
    A. Adenocarcinoma of oesophagus
    B. Adenocarcinoma of stomach
    C. Hodgkin's disease
    D. Soft tissue sarcomas

131. **Liver metastases of carcinoid tumour most fre-quently arise from a primary in the :**
    A. Appendix   B. Jejunum
    C. Ileum   D. Rectum

132. **Carcinoid syndrome occurs only if there is metastasis to :**
    A. Lung   B. Liver
    C. Brain   D. Bone

133. **Predisposing factors for colonic carcinomas are following except :**
    A. Familial polyposis   B. Gardner's syndrome
    C. Juvenile polyp   D. Chronic ulcerative colitis

134. **In carcinoma caecum, commonest surgery done is :**
    A. Total colectomy   B. Left hemicolectomy
    C. Right hemicolectomy   D. Ileostomy

135. **Which of the following is not peritoneal tumour?**
    A. Lipoma   B. Sarcoma
    C. Enterogenous cyst D. Ganglioneuroma

Ans.	127. C	128. A	129. B	130. C	131. C	132. B
	133. C	134. C	135. C			

136. At least 50% of the carcinomas of the colon are found in the :
    A. Sigmoid region   B. Caecum
    C. Splenic flexure   D. Transverse colon

137. The malignant tumour of the colon that most frequenlty occurs with ulcerative colitis is :
    A. Villous adenoma   B. Carcinoid
    C. Adenocarcinoma   D. Squamous cell carcinoma

138. The commonest retroperitoneal tumour is :
    A. Lymphosarcoma   B. Liposarcoma
    C. Pheochromocytoma   D. Neuroblastoma

139. True about intestinal lymphoma is :
    A. Most commonly found in jejunum
    B. May follow idiopathic malabsorption and steatorhoea
    C. Pain and constipation are chief complaints
    D. May be associated with pulm. and tricuspid stenosis

140. Colonic Carcinoma is associated with :
    A. Fatty food   B. Silicon
    C. PVC   D. Steel

141. Umbilical adenoma is most often a :
    A. Completely obliterated vitello intestinal duct
    B. Partially obliterated vitello intestinal duct
    C. Complete patent vitello intestinal duct
    D. Infection of umbilicus

142. Sacrococcygeal teratoma is commonly seen in :
    A. Males   B. Females
    C. Equality common   D. No predistable sex ratio

143. Most common tumour of duodenum is :
    A. Lymphoma   B. Leimyoma
    C. Villous tumor   D. Adenocarcinoma

144. Villous tumors of the gastrointestinal tract are least common in :
    A. Oesophagus   B. Duodenum
    C. Caecum   D. Rectum

145. The commonest presentation of adenoma of small intestine is :
    A. Intussuception   B. Intestinal bleeding
    C. Vomiting   D. Loss of appetite

146. The adenomatous polypi of large bowel are most often situated in :
    A. Ascending colon   B. Transverse colon
    C. Descending colon   D. Sigmoid colon

Ans.	136. A	137. C	138. A	139. B	140. A	141. B
	142. B	143. D	144. A	145. A	146. D	

147. **Umbilical granuloma is :**
    A. Infected umbilical cicatrix
    B. Adenoma
    C. Obliterated vitellointestinal duct
    D. Hydrocele

148. **In Jejunum, most common malignant tumor is :**
    A. Adenocarcinoma   B. Lymphosarcoma
    C. Carcinoid   D. Peutz Jeghers syndrome

149. **Scar carcinoma is common in :**
    A. TB pneumoconiosis   B. Interstitial fibrosis
    C. Pneumoconiosis   D. Pulmonary infarction

150. **Malignant potential is rare in following except :**
    A. Peutz Jeghers syndrome
    B. Adenomatous polyp
    C. Hamartomatous polyp
    D. Familial Adenomatous polyposis

151. **The least malignant form of carcinma colon is :**
    A. Annular   B. Tubular
    C. Ulcerative   D. Califlower

152. **Which of the following is not true about resberry tumour of umbilicus ?**
    A. Tumour of infant age group
    B. Rich in goblet cells
    C. Treatment in early stages consists of tying of ligature around it
    D. Arises from the skin near umbilicus

153. **Tratment of choice for Stage III a Hodgkins lymphoma :**
    A. Chemotherapy
    B. Radiotherapy
    C. Combination of chemotherapy and Radiotherapy
    D. Excision

154. **The most definitive indication of malignant transformation of a benign polyp of colon :**
    A. Infiltration of fibrous core
    B. Infilteation of base of polyp
    C. Ulceration at the tip of polyp
    D. Lymphatic permeation

155. **Tumor marker for colonic cancer is :**
    A. CEA   B. AFP
    C. HCG   D. Alpha antitrypsin

Ans.	147. A	148. A	149. D	150. B	151. D	152. D
	153. B	154. A	155. A			

156. The most common abdominal tumour in a child is :
    A. Embryoma of the kidney (Wilm's tumour)
    B. Neuroblastoma
    C. Malignant melanoma
    D. Benign sacrococcygeal teratoma

157. Sigmoid carcinoma with acute intestinal obstruction, treatment of choice :
    A. Proximal colostomy
    B. Resection and end-to-end-anastomosis
    C. Paul-Mickulicz operation
    D. Temporary colostomy

158. Surgery in not a treatment for :
    A. Lymphoma   B. Neuroblastoma
    C. Carcinoma colon   D. Carcinoma stomach

159. Pancreaticoduodenectomy is the treatment of choice for :
    A. Duodenal carcinoma
    B. Pancreatic carcinoma
    C. Gall Bladder Carcinoma
    D. Gastric carcinoma

160. A patient operated for carcinoma colon 4 months back now presents with a 2cm solitary mass in the liver. The best line of management is :
    A. Radiotherapy   B. Radiofrequency ablation   .
    C. Resection   D. CT scan

161. Constricting type of colonic carcinoma is seen in :
    A. Left colon   B. Right colon
    C. Transverse colon   D. Caecum

162. Which one of the following is not considered as precancerous lesion for carcinoma of the large bowel :
    A. Familial intestinal polyposis
    B. Vilious adenoma
    C. Chronic ulcerative colitis
    D. Peutz-Jegher's polyposis

163. All the following statements regarding malignant potential of colo-rectal polyps are true except :
    A. Polyps of familial polyposis coli could invariably undergo malignant change
    B. Pseudopolyps of ulcerative colitis has high risk of malignancy
    C. Villous adenoma is associated with high risk of malignancy
    D. Juvenile polyps has little or no risk

Ans. 156. B   157. C   158. A   159.A   160. C   161. A   162. D
      163. B

164. **All of the following are significant risk factors for colonic carcinoma in an adenomatous poly except?**
   A. Pedunculated polyp   B.   Villous histology
   C. Size > 2 cms   D.   Atypia

165. **The structures removed, while carrying out radical gastrectomy for a 2x2 cm antral adenocarcinoma, would include the following except :**
   A. Distal 2/3 of stomach with a centimetre cuff of duodenum
   B. Lesser and greater omentum
   C. Lymph nodes along left and right gastric common hepatic and splenic arteries
   D. Spleen

166. **A 1 cm x 1 cm squamous cell carcinoma of anal canal is best treated initially by :**
   A. Abdominoperineal resection
   B. Localised resection followed by irradiation
   C. Proximal colostomy followed by interstetial in adiation
   D. Chemo-radiotherapy

167. **Distal clearance in surgery for carcinoma rectum is :**
   A. 2 cm   B.   5 cm
   C. 10 cm   D.   8 cm

168. **To diagnose rectal growth, important procedure is :**
   A. PR examination   B.   Sigmoidoscopy
   C. Ba enema   D.   Ultrasound

169. **Rectal polyposis lead to loss of :**
   A. Na   B.   K
   C. Mg   D.   Ca

170. **After anterior resection of Ca rectum, the viability of rectal stump is determined by :**
   A. Superior mesenteric artery
   B. Inferior mesentric artery
   C. External iliac artery
   D. Internal iliac artery

171. **An elderly patient has been admitted with history of bleeding per retum. Rectal examination revealed a growth at a distance of 2 cm from the anal verge. The correct treatment will be :**
   A. Excision of the growth
   B. Abdomino-perineal resection
   C. Radiotherapy
   D. Chemotherapy

Ans.	164. A	165. D	166. D	167. A	168. A	169. B
	170. B	171. B				

172. **Regarding Rectal carcinoma the following statements are true except :**
    A. Adenomas and papillomas are pre cancerous conditions
    B. Local spread occurs circumferentially rather than longitudinally
    C. Lymphatic spread from Carcinoma of Rectum above the peritoneal reflection occurs almost exclusively in an upward direction
    D. Stage-D in the Duke's classification was originally described by Duke
    E. Bleeding is the earliest and most constant symptom

173. **In Duke's classification, B2 indicates :**
    A. Wall involvement including the muscularis
    B. Node involvement
    C. Distant metastasis to liver
    D. Local periodic fat invasion
    E. None of the above

174. **All of the following are characteristics of villous adenoma of rectum, except :**
    A. Large sessile growth
    B. Diarrhoea
    C. Rectal bleeding
    D. Frequent diagnosis by sigmoidoscopy
    E. Hyperkalaemia

175. **Common early presentation of carcinoma rectum is :**
    A. Pain
    B. Bleeding
    C. Increasing constipation
    D. Alternate constipation and diarrhoea

176. **Carcinoma of the rectum is characterized by following except :**
    A. Is squamous-celled
    B. Can occur in youth
    C. Causes bleeding which is slight in amount
    D. Simulates internal haemorrhoids

177. **"Cherry tumour" is a term for :**
    A. Metastatic polyp in rectum
    B. Pseudopolyp in sigmoid colon
    C. Juvenile polyp in rectum
    D. Adenomatous polyp in stomach

178. **Prognosis in cancer rectum is assessed by :**
    A. Size of tumour   B. Histological grading
    C. Site of tumour   D. Sex of the patient

Ans.	172. C	173. A	174. E	175. B	176. A	177. C
	178. B					

179. False statement regarding anal carcinoma is :
A. Is a epidermoid variety of carcinoma
B. Radiotherapy is given
C. Spreads to inguinal LN
D. Surgery is contraindicated

180. Match List I with List II and select the correct answer :

List I   List II
(Methods of treatment (Indications)
of carcinoma rectum)

A. Anterior resection   1. Carcinoma rectum causing intestinal obstruction
B. Hartman's procedure 2/3 rectum   2. Carcinoma of upper
C. Abdomino perineal   3. Carcinoma of lower 1/3 rd rectum
D. Palliative colostomy   4. Carcinoma rectum in an aged patient

	A	B	C	D
A.	3	1	2	4
B.	2	4	3	1
C.	2	1	3	4
D.	3	4	2	1

181. Villous polyps of rectum manifest with :
A. Bleeding PR
B. Mucus diarrhoea with hypokalaemia
C. Prolapsed rectum
D. Obstruction

182. Wrong about carcinoma Anus :
A. Squamous cell carcinoma
B. Spreads to Inguinal lymph nodes
C. Radiosensitive
D. Surgery contraindicated

183. Common type of carcinoma involving the anus is :
A. Melanoma
B. Adenocarcinoma
C. Transitional cell carcinoma
D. Epidermoid carcinoma

184. Malignant tumours of the anus is characterized by following except :
A. Include baseloid tumours
B. Primarily spread to the inferior mesenteric lymph nodes
C. May be treated by radiotherapy
D. Simulate anal fissure

Ans.	179. D	180. C	181. B	182. D	183. D	184. B

185. **Delorme's operation used in :**
 A. Rectal prolapse   B. Fistula-in-ano
 C. Fissure-in-ano   D. Rectum carcinoma

186. **Tumor presenting 3 cm from anal rogion is treated by :**
 A. Ant. resection of rectum
 B. ADR
 C. Chemoradiation
 D. Chemotherapy only

187. **The treatment of choice for cancer of the anal canal is :**
 A. Radiation
 B. Abdomino perineal resection
 C. Chemo-radiation
 D. Surgery and radiation

188. **A 50 yr old male, working as a hotel cook, has four dependent family members. He has been diagnosed with an early stage squamous cell cancer of anal canal. He has more than 60% chances of cure. The best treatment option is :**
 A. Abdomino-perineal resection
 B. Combined surgery and radiotherapy
 C. Combined chemotherapy and radiotherapy
 D. Chemotherapy alone

189. **The most common 'surgical' cause for bleeding per rectum in infants and children is due to :**
 A. Hemorrhoids   B. Intussusception
 C. Rectal polyp   D. Portal hypertension

190. **Regarding the carcinoid tumor of the rectum, which one of the following is not correct ?**
 A. It presents as an ulcer of the rectal mucosa
 B. Large carcinoid tumors are malignant
 C. Local excision of the tumor may be sufficient treatment for small (<2 cm) early tumors
 D. Carcinoid syndrome is rare

191. **For a rectal carcinoma at 5 cms from the anal verge the best acceptable operation is?**
 A. Anterior resection
 B. Abdomino-perineal resection
 C. Posterior resection
 D. Local resection

Ans.	185. A	186. C	187. C	188. C	189. C	190. A
	191. B					

192. **X-ray finding in metastatic carcinoma to mesentery and gut are all except :**
   A. Folds are angulated in their tips
   B. Thinning of bowel wall
   C. There will be oedema
   D. Immediate adjoining valvulae may appear spiked
   E. If metastasis invades, the mucosa ulceration produced

193. **X-ray features of lymphoma of stomach are all except :**
   A. Broad ulceration
   B. Moderate rigidity
   C. Perstalsis remain undisturbed
   D. Fingerprint impression pattern due to diffuse intramural invasion

194. **Widening of the C—loop in X-ray is diagnostic of :**
   A. Chronic pancreatitis
   B. Carcinoma head of pancreas
   C. Periampullary carcinoma
   D. Calculi in the ampula of Vater

195. **Most sensitive investigation of pancreatic carcinoma is :**
   A. Angiography   B. ERCP
   C. Ultrasound   D. CT Scan

196. **Best investigation for small bowel tumor is :**
   A. Enteroclysis
   B. Barium meal follow through
   C. Ultrasound
   D. CT

197. **Liver metastasis from G.I tract can sonographically present as :**
   A. Highly Echogenic
   B. Less Echogenic
   C. Hypoechoic
   D. Diffuse distortion of liver parenchyma

198. **In a child, most common cause of abdominal mass with calcification is :**
   A. Neuroblastoma   B. Bladder stone
   C. Wilm's tumor   D. Pulm Koch's

Ans.	192. B	193. C	194. B	195. D	196. A	197. A
	198. A					

GENITOURINARY SYSTEM

1. **When a 56 years old nulliparous, obese, diabetic lady comes with postmenopausal bleeding, the probable diagnosis is :**
   A. Granulosa cell tumour
   B. Carcinoma cervix
   C. Endometrial carcinoma
   D. Dysfunctional uterine bleeding

2. **Germ cell tumours of ovary are all except :**
   A. Dermoid cyst   B. Dysgerminoma
   C. Granulosa cell tumor D. None of the above

3. **The treatment of choice for recurrent endometrial carcinoma is**
   A. Irradiation   B. Surgical excision
   C. Mitomycin   D. Prosgestogens

4. **In carcinoma of cervix with spread to lateral pelvic walls, treatment of choice is :**
   A. Surgery   B. Chemotherapy
   C. Radiotherapy   D. Intracavitory radiotherapy

5. **Investigations for carcinoma cervix in the early stages are following except :**
   A. Surface biopsy
   B. Ultrasound
   C. Colposcopic guided biopsy
   D. Schiller's test

6. **Treatment of carcinoma cervix stage 3 B is :**
   A. Radiotherapy
   B. Chemotherapy
   C. Surgery
   D. Radiotherapy and chemotherapy

7. **Most common cause of suburethral metastasis :**
   A. Endometrial Ca   B. Cervical Ca
   C. Choriocarcinoma   D. Vaginal C

8. **A 30 years old female, G4, P1 on colposcopy was found to have carcinoma cervix. Manage-ment of choice is :**
   A. Cauterization
   B. Hysterectomy
   C. Termination and operation after 1 month
   D. Pregnancy to continue and operation after delivery

Ans.	1. C	2. C	3. D	4. C	5. B	6. A
	7. B	8. D				

9. **Fundal myomas commonly present as :**
   A. Inversion of uterus
   B. Dysmenorrhoea
   C. Urinary retention
   D. Menorrhagia

10. **In papillary adenocarcinoma of the uterine cornua, lympahtic spread will occur to —— nodes :**
    A. Internal iliac
    B. External iliac
    C. Inguinal
    D. Paraaortic

11. **Commonest complication of cryotherapy for carcinoma cervix in situ is :**
    A. Hemorrhage
    B. Persistant watery discharge
    C. Cervical stenosis
    D. Ulceration

12. **Metrorhagia in fibroid indicates :**
    A. Pregnancy
    B. Ovarian tumor
    C. Ulceration of submucus fibroid
    D. Twisting

13. **Ca endometrium with superficial inguinal LN is :**
    A. Stage I
    B. Stage II
    C. Stage III
    D. Stage IV

14. **A patient with 10 weeks pregnancy has an ovarian cyst of 6X4 inches. The treatment of choice is :**
    A. Removal of cyst at 14 weeks
    B. Terminate pregnancy and cyst removal
    C. Cesarean section at terms and removal of cyst
    D. Removal at puerperium

15. **The treatment of choice in a 56 year old woman with endometrial cancer is :**
    A. Irradiation
    B. Wertheim's hystrectomy
    C. Pan hystrectomy
    D. Irradiation and later panhysterectomy

16. **A case of carcinoma cervix presenting with persistent cough, distended abdomen, retention of urine, has :**
    A. Uraemia
    B. Intestinal obstruction
    C. Concealed haemorrhage
    D. Carcinoma extending into uterus

17. **Which of the following is false about fibroid :**
    A. Usually malignant
    B. Rare before 20 years
    C. Usually asymptomatic
    D. More common in nulliparous

Ans.	9. A	10. A	11. B	12. C	13. D	14. A
	15. C	16. A	17. A			

18. **In Dysplasia of Cx, following are seen except :**
   A. Pleomorphism
   B. Mitotic figure
   C. Loss of polarity
   D. Break in basement membrane
19. **Sarcoma Botyroides is mostly seen in :**
   A. Neonates   B. Children under 2 years
   C. Adults   D. Post menopausal
20. **The treatment of leukoplaqia of the vulva :**
   A. Irradiation   B. Simple vulvectomy
   C. Radical vulvectomy D. Estrogen cream
21. **Treatment of sarcoma boytroides is :**
   A. Irradiation   B. Total vaginectomy
   C. Radical hystrectomy D. B and C
22. **Endocervical involvement in endometrium is best diagnosed by :**
   A. Endocervical curretage B. CT
   C. MRI   D. Transvaginal USG
23. **True about dermoid is :**
   A. < 5% malignant
   B. Bilateral in 50%
   C. Common inmenopausal females
   D. All of the above
24. **The treatmentof choice in a full term lady with carcinoma cervix infilterating   walls is :**
   A. Vaginal caesarea B. Lower section caesarean
   C. Classical caesarean D. None of the above
25. **Consider the following statements about the condom :**
   It gives protection against
   1. Carcinoma cervix
   2. Carcinoma vulva
   3. Herpes simplex genitalis
   Of these statements
   A. 1 and 3 are correct B. 1 and 2 are correct
   C. 2 and 3 are correct D. 1, 2 and 3 are correct
26. **The most common type of ovarian tumor is :**
   A. Dermoid
   B. Pseudomucinous Cystadenoma
   C. Fibroma
   D. Cystadenocarcinoma

Ans.	18. D	19. B	20. B	21. D	22. A	23. A
	24. C	25. A	26. B			

27. **Call-Exner bodies are seen in :**
    A. Theca cell tumor   B. Fibromas
    C. Granulosa cell tumor D. None of the above

28. **Most common mallignancy of the Vagina :**
    A. Adeno Ca   B. Lymphoma
    C. Squamous Cell CA   D. Adeno-Cystic

29. **Ca cervix stage III B, Treatment of choice is :**
    A. Chemotherapy   B. Radiotherapy
    C. Surgery   D. Surgery + Radiotherapy

30. **True about Epidermid tumor :**
    A. Develops from epithelium
    B. Conain sebaceous material
    C. Always 10 cm in size
    D. Usually malignant

31. **Carcinoma cervix is commonest at :**
    A. Portio
    B. Endocervix
    C. Erosion
    D. Squamocolumnar junction

32. **Chorio carcinoma occur in :**
    A. H. mole   B. Fibroids
    C. Fibroma   D. Fibroids red degeneration

33. **Commonest malignancy in women in India is :**
    A. Ca-breast   B. Oral Ca
    C. Ca-cervix   D. Ovarian Ca

34. **The cause of virilizing adrenal hyperplasia is :**
    A. A defect in cortisol synthesis
    B. A defect in ACTH synthesis
    C. A defect in Androgen synthesis
    D. All of the above
    E. None of the above

35. **The extrauterine sites for occurrence of fibroids are except :**
    A. Round ligament   B. Inguinal canal
    C. Infundibulum   D. Ampulla

36. **Diagnosis of small polyps of uterus is by :**
    A. Curettage   B. Uterine sound
    C. Hystereoscopy   D. Hysterography

37. **Growth of a uterine myoma in a post menopausal patient suggests**
    A. Fatty degeneration   B. Cystic degeneration
    C. Calcareous degeneatio D. Sarcomatous change
    E. Hyaline degeneration

Ans.	27. C	28. C	29. B	30. A	31. D	32. A
	33. C	34. A	35. D	36. C	37. D	

38. Uterine sarcomas constitute about ——— % of all malignant growths of uterus :
    A. 5   B. 10
    C. 15   D. 20
    E. 25

39. The treatment of choice of sarcoma of uterus is :
    A. Total hysterectomy
    B. Total hysterectomy with bilateral salpingo-oophorectomy
    C. Radiotherapy
    D. B followed by C
    E. Chemotherapy

40. Chief characteristic of grape like sarcoma of cervix include all of the following except :
    A. Grape like vesicles
    B. A mixed mesodermal tumour which often contains cartilage striated muscle fibres, glands and fat
    C. Similar tumours are known to develop in vagina and body of uterus
    D. Metastasis develops rapidly and recurrence follows their removal
    E. Tumour is known for its common occurence

41. The peak age incidence of carcinoma of the endometrium is :
    A. 35 yrs   B. 40 yrs
    C. 45 yrs   D. 50 yrs
    E. 55 yrs

42. Carcinoma of the endometrium is most likely to occur in :
    A. Nulliparous   B. Uniparous
    C. Biparous   D. Multiparous
    E. Not related with parity

43. Submucous myoma of the uterus if symptomatic, most possible causes :
    A. Lower abdominal pain
    B. Constipation
    C. Unilateral hydronephrosis
    D. Excessive menstrual loss
    E. None of the above

44. The commonest degeneration occurring in uterine myoma is :
    A. Fatty degeneration
    B. Cystic degeneration
    C. Calcareous degeneration
    D. Hyaline degeneration
    E. Sarcomatous degeneration

Ans.   38. A   39. D   40. E   41. E   42. A   43. D
      44. D

45. Surgical treatment for asymptomatic uterine   myoma is indicated if :
   A. The myoma is pedunculated
   B. Tumour is larger than the size of 3 months pregnancy
   C. Diagnosis is uncertain
   D. All of the above
   E. None of the above

46. Which of the following types of myoma produces maximum symptoms
   A. Cervical   B. Submucous
   C. Intramural   D. Subscrous
   E. Pedunculated

47. Uterine myomas most likely originate from :
   A. Muture muscle cells
   B. Immature striated muscle
   C. Endothelium of vessels
   D. Immature smooth muscle
   E. Any of the above

48. Intramural uterine myomas most often cause menorrhagia due to :
   A. Pressure necrosis
   B. Rupture into endometrial cavity
   C. Secondary degeneration
   D. Inhibition of uterine contractility
   E. All of the above

49. The uncommon change to occur in a myoma is :
   A. Calcification   B. Red degeneration
   C. Myxomatous change D. Hyaline change

50. Myomas is associated with which endometrial pattern commonly :
   A. Follicular   B. Proliferative
   C. Secretary   D. None

51. The best time to remove an ovarian tumour in pregnancy is :
   A. Ist Trimester
   B. 16-18 weeks
   C. After 20 weeks
   D. Any time ovarian tumour is diagnosed

52. A very early case of carcinoma cervix usually presents with :
   A. Postcoital bleeding   B. Cervical discharge
   C. Pain   D. Abnormal bleeding
   E. Symptomless

Ans.	45. D	46. B	47. D	48. D	49. C	50. B
	51. B	52. D				

53. **Which is not a tumor in reproductive age group :**
   A. Ca ovary   B. Ca vulva
   C. Ca cervix   D. Ca uterus
54. **The commonest cause of death in carcinoma of cervix is :**
   A. Infection   B. Bleeding
   C. Uraemia   D. Cachexia
   E. Distant metastasies
55. **The most reliable procedure used to evaluate the patient with an abnormal cytologic smear but normal appearing cervix is :**
   A. Multiple punch biopsis
   B. Cold knife conization
   C. Cold knife conization and D and C
   D. D and C alone
   E. None of the above
56. **The most effective screening technique for detecting carcinoma in situ of cervix is :**
   A. Pap smear   B. Schiller's stain
   C. Lugol's stain   D. Examination of dried smear
   E. None of the above
57. **Which of the following is Schiller positive ?**
   A. Erosion   B. Ectropion
   C. Carcinoma cervix D. Leukoplakia
   E. All of the above
58. **Fibroids in pregnancy should be removed :**
   A. In pregnancy
   B. During caseerean section
   C. In the early pueperium
   D. Should not be removed
59. **Epidermidisation is :**
   A. A malignant condition B. A premalignant condition
   C. A benign lesion   D. None of the above
60. **Which of the following is not true about mucous polypi of cervix ?**
   A. They are usually pea sized
   B. The surface in smooth
   C. They bleed easily on touch
   D. They are hard
   E. They are usually pedunculated
61. **All of the following are true about Ca cervix except :**
   A. Screening test does not detect
   B. Coital bleeding early sign

Ans.	53. B	54. C	55. C	56. A	57. E	58. D
	59. C	60. D	61. A			

C. Herpes virus cancerous

D. Multiple partners predisposition

62. **Amenable to chemotherapy is :**
    A. Choriocarcinoma   B. Melanoma
    C. Dermoid cyst   D. Teratocarcinoma

63. **Aetiological agent hypothesized for carcinoma cervix is :**
    A. Herpes simplex I   B. Herpes simplex II
    C. Hepatitis virus   D. Chlamydia trachomatis

64. **Treatment of single large fibroid in a 45 years old female is :**
    A. Hysterectomy   B. Myomectomy
    C. Observe till menopaus D. Oral pills

65. **Still the first and the main treatment of ovarian tumour is :**
    A. Surgery   B. Chemotherapy
    C. Radiotherapy   D. Immunotherapy

66. **Commonest malignancy of the body of the uterus is :**
    A. Adenocanthoma   B. Squamous cell carcinoma
    C. Sarcoma   D. Adenocarcinoma

67. **Regarding fallopian tube tumour which is wrong ?**
    A. Adenocarcinoma
    B. 50% of people usually nulliparous
    C. Extremely rare
    D. Usually unilateral

68. **Classical Meig's syndrome is associated with which ovarian tumor :**
    A. Fibroma   B. Cystadenoma
    C. Thecoma   D. Granulosa cell tumour

69. **Commonest benign ovarian tumor is :**
    A. Lipoma   B. Fibroadenoma
    C. Paget's disease   D. Melanoma

70. **Hela cell line is associated with :**
    A. Carcinoma endometrium   B. Cancer cervix
    C. Carcinoma vulva   D. Ovarian carcinoma

71. **Brenner's tumor is always :**
    A. Brown   B. Yellow
    C. Blue   D. Red

72. **Among the various presenting symptoms, patients with ovarian malignancy which one of the following manifestations is the most common ?**
    A. Abnormal vaginal bleeding
    B. Gastrointestinal symptoms
    C. Abdominal distention and/or discomfort
    D. Urinary complaints (pressure frequency)

Ans.	62. A	63. B	64. C	65. A	66. D	67. B
	68. A	69. B	70. B	71. B	72. C	

73. **Roughly what percentage of patients with metastatic epithelial ovarian cancer will be benefitted by treatment with an alkylating agent ?**
   A. Less than 10 per cent B. 25 to 49 per cent
   C. 50 to 74 per cent   D. 75 to 89 per cent
   E. More than 90 per cent

74. **Severe dysplasia on Pap smear, Next step is :**
   A. Colloscopic directed biopsy
   B. Schilter's test + Multiple punch biopsy
   C. Cone biopsy
   D. Fractional curettage

75. **A 15 year old girl who had retention of urine and pain at the time of menstruation is suffering from :**
   A. Cervical fibroid   B. Sarcoma butyroides
   C. Endometriosis externa D. Adenomyosis

76. **Myomectomy is usually done ——— month after caesarean :**
   A. 1   B. 3
   C. 6   D. 12

77. **A patient after delivery develops amenorrhoea, anovulation, libido and absence of lactation. She has :**
   A. Ovarian tumour   B. Sheehan's syndrome
   C. Pituitary tumour   D. Polycystic ovary

78. **Treatment of malignant ovarian tumour is :**
   A. Chemotherapy
   B. Radiotherapy
   C. Surgery (debulking)
   D. Debulking + radiotherapy

79. **About Krukenberg tumor, all are true   except :**
   A. Maintains ovary shape
   B. Large cystic
   C. Bilateral
   D. Usually from stomach

80. **Ovarian tumour causing procecious puberty is :**
   A. Arrhenoblastoma   B. Dysgerminoma
   C. Granulosa cell tumour D. Gynandroblastoma

81. **About chorio-carcinoma, wrong is :**
   A. Maternal tissue origin
   B. Increased HCG
   C. Incomplete abortion is the differential diagnosis
   D. Haemoptysis maximally present

Ans.	73. C	74. A	75. C	76. C	77. B	78. D
	79. B	80. C	81. A			

82. A patient 30 yr old, with 2 children, on pap smear stage III CIN.
     What is the next line of managment :
     A. Repeat smear
     B. Schillers test
     C. Colpomicroscopic biopsy
     D. Hysterectomy

83. A CaCx patient, develops unilateral renal shut down or hydrone-
     phosis - what is the staging of this disease :
     A. Stage II A   B.   Stage III B
     C. Stage IV A   D.   Stage IV B

84. A 65-year-old female with anorexia, ascites, mass arising from
     pouch of Douglas and it is felt with uterus. Diagnosis is :
     A. Malignant ovarian tumour
     B. Fibroid
     C. Endometriosis
     D. Adenocarcinoma uterus

85. Vulvar cancer occurs commonly in the age of group of :
     A. 30-40 year   B.   40-50 years
     C. 60-70 years   D.   Any age group

86. The ovarian tumour diagnosed after delivery should be removed :
     A. Immediately after the 3rd stage
     B. Within 48 hours of delivery
     C. After one week
     D. Only after 6 weeks

87. Endometrial Ca, lymph node spread is not to :
     A. Paraortic   B.   Inguinal
     C. Inferior mesentric   D.   Pre sacral

88. Herpes virus type II infection of cervix can lead to :
     A. Chronic cervicitis   B.   Carcinoma cervix
     C. Cervical erosion   D.   P.I.D.

89. The most malignant veriety of carcinoma cervix is :
     A. Spinal cell carcinoma
     B. Spindle cell carcinoma
     C. Transitional cell carcinoma
     D. Adeno carcinoma

90. The incidence of stump carcinoma is :
     A. 0.5%   B.   1%
     C. 1.5%   D.   2%

Ans.	82. D	83. B	84. A	85. C	86. B	87. C
	88. B	89. B	90. B			

91. In carcinoma endometrium if the length of the uterine cavity > 8 cm it is :
    A. Stage I a   B. Stage Ib
    C. Stage O   D. Stage IIb

92. The incidence of vaginal vault recurrence in carcinoma enodmetrium is :
    A. 10-15 %   B. 5-10 %
    C. < 5%   D. None of the above

93. The most common complication of subserous myoma is :
    A. Capsule rupture   B. Torsion
    C. Inversion   D. Inflammation

94. Fibromyoma becomes painful if it undergoes :
    A. Red degeneration   B. Haemorrhage
    C. Torsion   D. Sarcomatous change
    E. All of the above

95. Degeneration of the myomata is more likely to start from :
    A. Centre   B. Periphery
    C. From any portion   D. None of the above

96. Which of the following is classified under neutral mesenchymoma ?
    A. Dysgerminoma   B. Brenner tumour
    C. Granulosa cell tumour   D. Theca cell tumour
    E. Luteoma

97. A tumour having the characteristic of both the granulosa cell tumour and the arrhenoblastoma is known as :
    A. Dysgerminoma   B. Luteoma
    C. Hilus cell tumour   D. Gynandroblastoma
    E. Krukenberg tumour

98. Femimising mesenchymoma may include :
    A. Granulosa cell tumour   B. Luteoma
    C. Theca cell tumour   D. All of the above
    E. None of the above

99. Which of the following is not true about cystoma simplex (simple serous cystadenoma)?
    A. It is usually bilateral
    B. The tumour is unilocular
    C. The lining epithelium is single layered
    D. It contains a clear fluid
    E. Average size is about 10 cms in diamter

Ans.	91. B	92. A	93. B	94. E	95. A	96. A
	97. D	98. D	99. A			

100. Ovarian tumours regarded as representing forms of ovarian mullerianosis :
A. Simple serous cystadenoma + papillary serous cystadenoma
B. Fibromata + Sarcomata
C. Dermoid cysts + Struma ovarii
D. All of the above

101. Sarcomatous change in leiomyoma is less than :
A. 0.5%   B. 1%
C. 5%   D. 10%

102. Corpus luteum cysts are frequently found in :
A. Early pregnancy
B. Menopausal age
C. Post menopausal period
D. Prepubertal period
E. All of the above

103. Which of the following is not true about corpus luteum cysts ?
A. The wall is thin
B. They contain clear yellow fluid
C. They are usually pathological
D. The wall contains the normal convolutions
E. They rarely cause localising symptoms

104. In corpus luteum haematomata the blood is found in :

A. Theca interna layer
B. Granulosa lutein layer
C. Cavity of the corpus luteum
D. All of the above
E. None of the above

105. Which of the following is not true about granulosa-lutein cysts ?
A. Convolutions are present
B. They are thin walled
C. Well marked luteinization of both granulosa and theca interna cells
D. They are produced due to increased chorionic gonadotrophic hormone in the circulation
E. The large cystic ovary may undergo torsion

106. All of the following are tumours rising from the ovum, except :
A. Chorion epithelioma   B. Dermoid cysts
C. Fibromata   D. Solid teratoma

107. Non endocrine secreting tumor of ovary is :
A. Fibroma   B. Arrhenoblastoma
C. Gynandroblastoma D. Hilus cell tumour

Ans.	100. A	101. A	102. A	103. C	104. D	105. A
	106. C	107. A				

108. **In carcinoma cervix of the growth involves the upper third of vagina, it is staged as :**
    A. Ia   B. IIa
    C. IIb   D. IIIa

109. **Which of the following is not epithelial cell in origin :**
    A. Teratoma
    B. Brenner
    C. Serous cystadenoma carcinoma
    D. Pseudomucinous

110. **Red degeneration of fibroid is associated with :**
    A. Pregnancy   B. Aseptic infarction
    C. Thrombosis   D. Leukocytosis

111. **Endometrial caricinoma is usually associated with all except :**
    A. Diabetes mellitus   B. Hypertension
    C. Obesity   D. Multiparity

112. **A large cervical fibroid most commonly presents with :**
    A. Menorrhagia   B. Retention of urine
    C. Abdominal mass   D. Mass per vagina

113. **Endometrial carcinoma is diagnosed by :**
    A. Curettage and examination
    B. Exfoliative cytology
    C. Pap smear
    D. Hormone estimation

114. **The ovarian tumour that attains the largest size is :**
    A. Simple seous cystadenoma
    B. Papillary serous cystadenoma
    C. Pseudomucinous cystadenoma
    D. Brenner tumour

115. **Out of all ovarian neoplasms ovarian carcinoma comprises of :**
    A. 5-15%   B. 15-25%
    C. 25-35%   D. 35-45%

116. **Dermoid cyst have all the following characters except :**
    A. Cystic
    B. Teratogenous elements are immature
    C. Subdivision of ovarian teratoma
    D. May contain hair and sebaceous material
    E. May be combined with cystadenoma

117. **The treatment of choice for early invasive carcinoma vulva is :**
    A. Radical vulvectomy with lymphadenectomy
    B. Interstitial radium implantation followed by lymphadenectomy
    C. External radiation only
    D. Multi-drug chemotherapy

Ans.	108. D	109. A	110. A	111. D	112. B	113. A
	114. C	115. A	116. B	117. A		

118. **All of the following can be attributed to Arrheno-blastoma except for :**
A. A masculinising tumour
B. Origin in from adrenal rest cells
C. Recurrence rate after removal is 25%
D. Occur in patient from 20 to 30
E. Clinically starts as benign and follows with masculanization

119. **Inheritance is a major factor in :**
A. Endometrial Ca B. Cervical Ca
C. Both D. Neither

120. **Regarding the treatment of Cancer cervix in pregnancy all of the are correct, except :**
A. For carcinoma-in-situ, treatment is detered until the postpartum period
B. For more advanced cases, the disease should be treated without regard to the pregancy
C. If the pregnancy is beyond 28 weeks, baby can be delivered by Caesarean section
D. In cervical intra-epithelial elloplasia baby is usually delivered by caesarean section

121. **The best method of diagnosis of cancer cervix in ulcerative stage is by :**
A. Cervical smear B. Cervical biopsy
C. Colposcopy D. None of the above

122. **Carcinoma endometrium is frequenlty associated with :**
A. Postmenospausal bleeding
B. Pyometra
C. Endometrial polyp
D. All of the above
E. None of the above

123. **For mass screening of genital malignancy with Pap's smear, the smear is obtained from :**
A. Anterior vaginal fornix
B. Posterior vaginal fornix
C. Scraping from around the cervical os
D. Endometrial washings

124. **A 60 year old nullipara has Vaginal bleeding for a week. The most probable diagnosis is :**
A. Cancer cervix
B. Cancer vagina
C. Dysfunctional uterine bleeding
D. Cancer body uterus

| Ans. | 118. B | 119. A | 120. D | 121. B | 122. D | 123. B |
| | 124. D | | | | | |

125. **Endocrinal function is always present in the following ovarian neoplasms :**
    A. Brenner tumour
    B. Dysgerminoma
    C. Strauma ovarii
    D. All of the above

126. **The 'signet ring' type of epithelial cell scattered in a myxomatous stroma of the ovarian tumour is characteristic of :**
    A. Dysgerminoma
    B. Mesonephroma
    C. Embryonal cell carcinoma
    D. Kruckenberg's tumour

127. **The most useful diagnostic aid of carcinoma in situ :**
    A. Colposcopy
    B. Cervical smear study
    C. Punch biopsy
    D. Cone biopsy and serial study

128. **Premalignant lesion of the vulva is :**
    A. Kraurosis
    B. Leucoplakia
    C. Condyloma accuminate
    D. Localised scleroderma

129. **Vaginal bleeding in the age period over 60 years may be commonly caused by each of the following except :**
    A. Cervical carcinoma in situ
    B. Granulosa cell tumour of the ovary
    C. Uterine carcinoma
    D. Atrophic vaginitis
    E. All of the above

130. **Cervical dystocia is usually present at :**
    A. Level of external os
    B. Level of internal os
    C. Levl of isthmus
    D. Level of cervical canal

131. **Which type of fibroid is most prone to undergo sarcomatous changes :**
    A. 12th week
    B. 16th week
    C. 20th week
    D. 24th week

132. **In the body of uterus commonest type of myoma is :**
    A. Subserous
    B. Submucous
    C. Intramura
    D. All have equal incidence

133. **Bladder is usually affected in :**
    A. Intramural myoma
    B. Subserous myoma
    C. Submucous myoma
    D. Crevical myomas
    E. None of the above

Ans.	125. C	126. D	127. D	128. B	129. A	130. A
	131. D	132. C	133. D			

134. **Regarding aetiology of fibroid each of the following is true except :**
    A. Most common in women who are either sterile or have born only one child
    B. Tumour develops commonly after child birth
    C. An oestrogen dependent tumour
    D. Commonest in age group 35-45 yrs
    E. None of the above

135. **The growth of myoma is an oestrogen dependent phenomenon. This hypothesis is suggested by :**
    A. Enlarged hyperaemic ovaries
    B. The tumour becomes smaller after menopause
    C. Fairly frequent association of tumour with endometriosis and endometrial hyperplasia
    D. All of the above
    E. None of the above

136. **Virchow demonstrated that fibroids are essentially :**
    A. Myoma
    B. Leiomyoma
    C. Leimyosarcomas
    D. Fibromas
    E. None of the above

137. **Fibroids are common in which age group ?**
    A. 15-25 yrs
    B. 25-35 yrs
    C. 35-45 yrs
    D. 55-65 yrs

138. **Anatomically a myoma is characterised by all of the following, except :**
    A. All uterine myomas arise in myometrium
    B. The capsule consists of connective tissue which fixes the tumour to myometrium
    C. The vessels which supply the tumour lie in the capsule
    D. The middle part of the tumour has got richest blood supply
    E. Degenerations are commonest in middle part of tumour

139. **Lymphocytic infiltration amongst masses of large tumour cells is diagnostic of :**
    A. Brenner tumour
    B. Hillus cell tumour
    C. Dysgerminoma
    D. Dermoid tumor

140. **The treatment of choice for Grape like sarcoma of vagina is :**
    A. Total vaginectomy
    B. A+Radical hysterectomy
    C. A+chemotherapy
    D. Irradiation

141. **The microscopic features of leukoplakia vulva include :**
    A. Inflammatory infiltrate
    B. Hyperkeratosis
    C. Acanthosis
    D. All of the above
    E. None of the above

Ans.	134. B	135. D	136. B	137. C	138. D	139. C
	140. B	141. D				

142. The treatment of choice for carcinoma in situ in a patient of 35 years old, 3rd para :
    A. Conization
    B. Hysterectomy
    C. BSO + TAH
    D. Total hysterectomy with removal of cuff of vagina

143. Which of the following is the commonest site for beginning of the carcinoma of the cervix ?
    A. 3 O'clock and 9 O' clock
    B. 6 O' clock and 8 O'clock
    C. 9 O'clock and 10 O'clock
    D. 6 O' clock and 12 O' clock
    E. 4 O' clock and 8 O'clock

144. A 38 year old multipara has a report of carcinoma in situ of cervix returned on a biopsy specimen, the procedure which should be followed is :
    A. Hysterectomy   B. Full course of radiation
    C. Cryo surgery   D. Cold knife conization
    E. Colpomicroscopy

145. The stage of carcinoma of cervix is determined by :
    A. Physical examination   B. Exploratory laparatomy
    C. Biopsy   D. Staining techniques
    E. All of the above

146. The treatment of choice for carcinoma in situ of cervix is :
    A. Chemotherapy   B. Surgery
    C. Radiation   D. All of the above
    E. None of the above

147. Fibroids are associated with carcinoma endometrium in :
    A. 3%   B. 5%
    C. 10%   D. 15%

148. Ovarian secondaries characterized by mucin secretion may have their primary in :
    A. The breast   B. The stomach
    C. The gall bladder   D. All of the above

149. The commonest ovarian tumour found in children :
    A. Teratoma   B. Arrhenoblastoma
    C. Gynandroblastoma   D. Dysgerminoma
    E. Mesonephroma

Ans.	142. D	143. D	144. A	145. A	146. B	147. A
	148. D	149. A				

150. **Disontogenic ovarian neoplasm include all of the following except:**
    A. Theca tumours   B. Hilus tumour
    C. Arrhenoblastoma   D. Dysgerminoma
    E. Granulosa cell tumour

151. **Most common complication of ovarian cyst is :**
    A. Torsion   B. Malignant degeneration
    C. Suppuration   D. Rupture

152. **The surgery of choice for malignant ovarian tumour is :**
    A. Unilateral salphino-oophorectomy
    B. Bilateral salpingo-oophorectomy
    C. Unilateral salpingo-oophorectomy + total hysterectomy
    D. Total hysterectomy + Bilateral salpingo-oophorectomy

153. **All of the following may produce chorionic gonadotrophin, except :**
    A. Teratoma   B. Choriocarcinoma
    C. Dysgerminoma   D. Mesonephroma

154. **Attacks of flushing and cyanosis occur in which type of ovarian tumours ?**
    A. Struma ovarii
    B. Krukenberg tumour
    C. Arrhenoblastoma
    D. Carcinoid tumours of ovary
    E. Granulosa cell tumour

155. **Urethral caruncles are best treated by :**
    A. Electrocautery   B. Podophyllin
    C. Topical steroids   D. Excision

156. **Which of the following may be caused by granulosa cell tumour ?**
    A. Precocious puberty
    B. Amenorrhoea followed by prolonged bleeding in young patients
    C. Post menopausal bleeding
    D. All of the above

157. **Metastases from a granulosa cell tumour first involves :**
    A. The liver   B. The opposite ovary
    C. The mesentery   D. The mediastinum

158. **Theca cell tumour usually arises :**
    A. Before puberty
    B. Just after puberty
    C. Active reproductive lif
    D. After menopause

Ans.	150. B	151. A	152. D	153. D	154. D	155. D
	156. D	157. B	158. D			

159. An ovarian tumour showing large cells with large darkstaining nuclei, and almost translucent cytoplasm along with lymphocytic infiltrationa of the fibrous septa is diagnostic of :
   A. Dysgerminoma   B. Arrhenoblastoma
   C. Gynandroblastoma D. None of the above

160. Myxoma peritonei may follow rupture of a :
   A. Serous cyst adenoma
   B. Dermoid cyst
   C. Struma ovarii
   D. Pseudomucinous cystadenoma
   E. Arrhenoblastoma

161. Carcinoma Cervi involving upper 2/3 of vagina are classed as :
   A. IIA   B. IIB
   C. IIIA   D. IIIB

162. Carcinoma of fundus of uterus can spread to all the following lymph nodes except :
   A. Inguinal   B. Obturator
   C. Intenal iliac   D. Para-aortic

163. Among following most common type of Benign ovarian tumour during pregnancy is :
   A. Simple serous cystoid B. Mucinous cystoid
   C. Teratoma   D. Papillary Cystadenoma

164. Treatment of choice in a perimenopausal female with bleeding P/V due to multiple fibroids is :
   A. TAH   B. TAH with BSO
   C. Vaginal hysterectomy   D. Enucleation of fibroids

165. Chemotherapy is most useful in the treatment of Cancer of :
   A. Cervix   B. Ovary
   C. Uteus   D. Vulva

166. Vulval carcinoma metastasizes to which group of nodes ?
   A. Superficial inguinal nodes
   B. External iliac nodes
   C. Internal Iliac nodes
   D. Para-aortic nodes

167. Most common ovarian tumor to undergo torsion is :
   A. Pseudomucionous cystadenoma
   B. Papillary cystadenoma
   C. Dermoid cyst
   D. Mucinous cyst

Ans.	159. A	160. D	161. C	162. B	163. C	164. A
	165. B	166. A	167. A			

168. **In carcinoma cervix, prognosis depends on :**
    A. Staging   B. Lymphadenopathy
    C. Symptoms   D. All of the above

169. **One of the following shows features of ovarian mullenanosis :**
    A. Dermoid cyst   B. Serous cystoadenoma
    C. Brenner's tumor   D. Granulosa cell tumor

170. **Primary of Krukenberg tumor is found in ——— of stomach :**
    A. Lesser curvature   B. Cardia
    C. Fundus   D. Pylorus

171. **Hyaline degeneration in myomata most often causes :**
    A. Pain   B. Menorrhagia
    C. Oligomenorrhoea   D. None specific symptoms

172. **Poor prognosis of ovarian tumor is because of :**
    A. Inadequate diagnostic tests
    B. Inadequate treatment
    C. Silent early growth
    D. Inadequate investigation

173. **Risk of development of endometrial carcinoma is highest with which of the following ovarian tumour :**
    A. Granulosa cell tumor   B. Theca cell tumour
    C. Mucinous cystadenom   D. Serous cystadenoma

174. **All the following are the reasons for menorrhagia in a case of fibroid uterus except :**
    A. Endometrial hyperplasia
    B. Myohyperplasia
    C. Increased bleeding surface
    D. Low prostaglandin levels

175. **Alpha-feto protein is a most useful tumour marker in which of the following germ cell tumours :**
    A. Endodermal sinus tumor
    B. Choriocarcinoma
    C. Dysgerminoma
    D. Teratoma

176. **A patient comes with gravida 4, living with 22 weeks of pregnancy with carcinoma insitu. The treatment of choice is :**
    A. Conisation of the cervix
    B. MTP and hysterectomy
    C. MTP and radiotherapy
    D. Allow the baby to be born and then hysterrectomy

Ans.	168. D	169. B	170. D	171. D	172. C	173. A
	174. D	175. A	176. D			

177. A patient with carcinoma cervix who has completed radiotherapy comes with uraemia. The most common cause is :
   A. Bilateral ureter invasion
   B. Radiation nephritis
   C. Ureteric stenosis due to radiation
   D. Unconnected causes

178. Most important role of colposcopy in cancer detection programme lies in :
   A. Screening large population
   B. Confirmation of abnormal cytological smears
   C. Localisation of an abnormal area on the surface of cervix
   D. Diagnosis of dysplasia and cercinoma in situ of cervix

179. Virilising tumours of the ovary are :
   A. Arrhenoblastoma
   B. Adrenal tumours of the ovary
   C. Leydig cell tumour
   D. Gynandroblastoma
   E. All of the above

180. The patient is a 35-year old who has aborted twice at the 18th gestational week and she has complained or severe dysmenorrhea, hypermenorrhea, some increased vaginal discharge and spotting intermenstrually. On pelvic examination the uterus was slightly irregular, firm and enlarged to an 8 week gestatinal size. The impression is that she has leiomyomatous uterus. What type of uterine tumor is associated with these types of clinical presentations :
   A. Submucous leimyoma
   B. Intramural leiomyoma
   C. Subserosal leiomyoma
   D. Intraligamentary leiomyoma or (parasitic)
   E. None of the above

181. In which phase of menstrual cycle a fibroid uterus is most likely to cause retention of urine ?
   A. Proliferative phase
   B. Mid cycle
   C. Early secretory phase
   D. Late secretary and menstrual phase

182. Vulvar carcinoma with hypertension and DM. Treatment of choice is :
   A. Radiotherapy   B. Chemotherapy
   C. Surgery   D. Hormonal therapy

Ans.	177. A	178. D	179. E	180. A	181. A	182. C

183. **A woman with an asymptomatic fibroid uterus must be advised surgery if the size of the tumour is more than :**
    A. 8 weeks   B. 10 weeks
    C. 12 weeks   D. 14 weeks

184. **Adenocarcinoma of vagina is caused by :**
    A. Megestrol   B. Diethylstiboesterol
    C. Medroxyprogestrone D. Dydrogesterone

185. **The most appropriate management of a case of 14 weeks gestation with benign ovarian cyst is :**
    A. Conservative treatment
    B. Laparotomy after delivery
    C. Removal of cyst with elective LSCS at term
    D. Immediate laparotomy and cyst removal

186. **In a case of badly eroded cervix, if biopsy of a random site showed carinoma in situ, then the next logical step would be :**
    A. Cone biopsy   B. Panhystectomy
    C. Vaginal cytology   D. Schiller's test

187. **The treatment for a 60-year old lady with a right-sided benign ovarian tumour is :**
    A. Total abdominal hysterectomy
    B. Right salpingo-ovariotomy
    C. Total hysterectomy with bilateral salpingo-oophorectomy
    D. Ovarian cystectomy

188. **Which of the following statement regarding dermoid cyst are true:**
    I.   They are one of the commonest ovarian tumours in young women
    II. They are unilateral in 10% of cases
    III. Torsion or rupture may produce signs and symptoms of an acute abdomen
    IV. They are potenitally malignant
    Select the correct answer using the codes given below :
    A. I and II   B. I and III
    C. II and IV   D. I, III and IV

189. **A 40-year old woman is suffering from severe menorrhagia due to multiple fibroids. Her uterus is irregularly enlarged to 16 weeks pregnancy size. She has three living children. Which one of the following would be best suited for her :**
    A. Total abdominal hysterectomy with bilateral salpingo-oophorectomy
    B. Total abdominal hysterectomy
    C. Vaginal hysterectomy
    D. Total abdominal hysterectomy with unilateral salpingo-oophorectom

Ans.	183. C	184. B	185. D	186. A	187. C	188. D
	189. B					

190. Ovarian tumor before 20 years of age is :
    A. Germ cell tumor   B. Sex and tumor
    C. Epithelial tumor   D. Embryonal cell tumor

191. Diffuse hyperkeratosis or parakeratosis of the cervix is most often associated with :
    A. Carcinoma in situ III   B. DES exposure in utero
    C. Human papilloma virus   D. Menopause
    E. Uterine descensus

192. The single most common metastatic cancer in unselected inguinal lymph nodes is :
    A. Carcinoma of the anus and rectum
    B. Carcinoma of the ovary
    C. Cervical carcinoma
    D. Melanoma
    E. Vulvarcarcinoma

193. Most pelvic exenterations are performed for carcinoma of the :
    A. Bladder   B. Vulva
    C. Cervix   D. Prostate
    E. Rectosigmoid

194. Epitheloid mesothelioma is histologically similar to :
    A. Fibroma
    B. Malignant teratoma
    C. Mucinous adenocarcinoma
    D. Serous papillary adenocarcinoma
    E. Thecoma

195. The best overall method of determining whether a patient is free of ovarian cancer :
    A. Peritoneal CA 125
    B. Peritoneal cytology
    C. Peritoneal washing CA 125
    D. Second look surgery
    E. Serum CA 125

196. Ca cervix Ia1 is --------------mm depth :
    A. Below 3   B. Above 3
    C. Below 7   D. Above 7

197. The most common benign ovarian neoplasm during the second and third decade is :
    A. Serous cystadenoma   B. Mucinous cystadenoma
    C. Benign cystic teratoma D. Fibroma

Ans.	190. A	191. A	192. D	193. C	194. D	195. B
	196. A	197. C				

198. In her first cycle of low dose triphasic oral contraceptives, a patient is found to have a 40 mm follicle-like structure on day 23 of a 28 day cycle. An ultrasound one month previous was negative. The structure is most likely :

    A. Corpus luteum   B. Dermoid cyst
    C. Follicle cyst   D. Serous cystadenoma
    E. Unruptured follicle

199. True statements about leiomyomata uteri in pregnancy include all except :

    A. Elective myomectomy at cesarean deli-very may be safe in carefully chosen patients
    B. Only myomata that are pedunculated should be considered for removal
    C. Most leiomyoamt remain asymptomatic during pregnancy
    D. Most leiomyomata grow during pregnancy

200. The only normal tissue to express the tumor associated antigen TAG-72 :

    A. Breast   B. Colon
    C. Endometrium   D. Myometrium
    E. Ovary

201. A patient if found to have vulvar intraepithelial neoplasia on a hairy portion of her vulva. To what depth (mm) should laser ablation be used to maximize cure and preserve the function of th epilosebaccous   glands ?

    A. 1.0   B. 1.25
    C. 1.50   D. 1.75
    E. 2.0

202. In diagnosing a leiomyoma as benign, consideration should be given to all except :

    A. Menstrual cycle
    B. Number of mitoses per hpf
    C. Patient's age
    D. Size of myoma

203. A 30-years old develops red degeneration of uterine fibroid after delivery. The treatment should be :

    A. Antibiotics
    B. Rest only
    C. Hysterectomy
    D. Hysterectomy with bilateral oophrectomy

Ans.	198. E	199. D	200. C	201. E	202. D	203. B

204. Stage I carcinoma cervix refers to :
    A. Carcinoma in situ
    B. Carcinoma confined to cervix
    C. Ca confined to vagina
    D. Ca extending to pelvic walls

205. The incidence of metastasis in carcinoma cervix stage II :
    A. 5-10%   B. 15-20%
    C. 25-40%   D. 50-60%

206. Clear cell adenocarcinoma of the vagina and vaginal adenosis appear to be more common in the following group of women than in the general population :
    A. Nuns
    B. Prostitutes
    C. Women on oral contraceptives
    D. Women exposed prenatally to diethylstilboestrol

207. Which of the following tumours does not metastasize to ovary :
    A. Breast   B. Stomach
    C. Colon   D. Cervix

208. Tt of GN grade III in 40 year old female :
    A. Laser   B. Surgery
    C. Radiotherapy   D. Conisation

209. Marker in epithelial Ca ovary :
    A. HCG   B. AVP
    C. CA-125   D. Oestrogens

210. Pelvic masses associated with endometrial hyperplasia include all of the following except :
    A. Dysgeminoma   B. Thecoma
    C. Granulosa cell tumour   D. Polycystic ovaries

211. A 20-year old non-pregnant patient with normal menstrual history has persistent enlargement of the left ovary (7 cm). The most likely diagnosis is :
    A. Follicular cyst   B. Corpus luteum cyst
    C. Benign cystic teratoma   D. The ovary is removed

212. Treatment of choice in young lady with cervical intraepithelial Neoplasia, stage 3, who has not completed the family is :
    A. Hysterectomy   B. Observation
    C. Couterization   D. Radiation

213. For FIGO staging of Ca carvix, followng investiga-tions are required except :
    A. Chest X-ray   B. IVP
    C. Cystoscopy   D. Pelvic ultrasound

Ans.	204. B	205. D	206. D	207. A	208. A	209. C
	210. B	211. C	212. C	213. A		

214. Psammoma bodies are seen in following except :
A. Serous cystadenoma of ovary
B. Mucinous cystadenoma of ovary
C. Meningioma
D. Papillary Ca thyroid

215. State IB Ca body uterus is :
A. Limited to endometrium
B. < 1/2 depth of myometrium involved
C. > 1/2 depth of myometrium involved
D. All of the above

216. Ultrasound in post menopausal female can detect ovarian cancer of > 1.5 mm) in :
A. 20%   B. 30%
C. 60%   D. 80%

217. Ca vagina extending to lateral pelvic wall is stage :
A. I   B. II
C. III   D. IV

218. Tumor associated with pregnancy is :
A. Dysgerminoma   B. Luteal cell carcinoma
C. Teratoma   D. Arrhenoblastoma

219. A 51-year old nulliparous lady complains of heavy, prolonged, irregular bleeding for the past 6 months. On examination, she was obese, moderately hypertensive with a blood pres-sure of 160/100 mm of Hg. Her breasts were normal. Per speculum examination revealed a health and nulliparous cervix. On bimanual examination, the uterus felt bulky irregularly enlarged to 12 weeks size, anteverted and mobile and ovaries were not palpable. The first line of management in this case will be to :
A. Give progestogens
B. Do a fractional curettage and cervical biopsy
C. Do hysteroscopy followed by fractional curettage
D. Do hysterectomy straight away

220. Which of the following pairs are correctly matched ?
1. Cancer of cervix   — Irregular
2. Cancer of endometrium —Adenocarcinoma
3. Dysgerminoma   — Menopause
4. Cancer vulva   — Pruritus
Select the correct answer using the codes given below :
Codes :
A. 1 and 2   B. 2, 3 and 4
C. 1,2 and 4   D. 1,3 and 4

Ans.	214. B	215. B	216. A	217. C	218. B	219. C
	220. C					

221. **Ca-cervix stage II means :**
   A. Involvement of upper 1/3rd vagina
   B. Lesion limitted to cervix
   C. Involvement of pelvis
   D. All of the above

222. **In Ca-cervix stage III-B, treatment of choice is :**
   A. Total abdominal hysterectomy (TAH)
   B. TAH with radiotherapy
   C. External radiation + Intracavitory radiation
   D. Chemotherapy

223. **Which of the following are the risk factors for the development of endometrial carcinoma ?**
   1. Prolonged use of oral contraceptives
   2. Polycystic ovarian disease
   3. Late menopause
   4. Anovulatory DUB.
   Codes :
   A. 1,2 and 4   B. 1,2 and 3
   C. 1,3 and 4   D. 2,3 and 4

224. **Following are sex cord stromal tumours of ovary except :**
   A. Fibroma
   B. Granulosa theca cell tumour
   C. Sertoli Leydig cell tumour
   D. Brenner tumour

225. **Malignant ovarian tumour is associated with :**
   A. Rapid growth   B. Ascities
   C. Fixity of tumour   D. All of the above

226. **Carcinoma involving both the ovaries with rupture of the capsule and ascitic fluid cytology positive for malignant cells is of stage:**
   A. I   B. II
   C. III   D. IV

227. **Treatment of fibroid:**
   A. Laser myolysis   B. Myomectomy
   C. Radio freq. ablalion D. Uterine artery occlusion

228. **Feature in USG suggestive of ovarian malignancy is :**
   A. Papillary pattern   B. Septations
   C. Bllaterality   D. Clear flui

229. **The first step in the management of hirustism due to Stein-Leventhal syndrome is :**
   A. OCP   B. HCRH
   C. Spironolactone   D. Bromocriptine

Ans.	221. C	222. C	223. A	224. D	225. D	226. C
	227. A	228. A	229. A			

230. **The ideal treatment for metastatic choriocarcinoma in the lungs in a young women is :**
   A. Chemotherapy
   B. Surgery with radiation
   C. Surgery
   D. Wait & Watch

231. **The colposcopic features suggestive of malignancy are except :**
   A. Condyloma
   B. Papillary process
   C. Punctation
   D. White epithelium

232. **In prolapse of cervix, decubitus ulcer is due to :**
   A. Trauma
   B. Venous congestion
   C. Friction
   D. Intercourse

W233. **Following are seen in granulosa cell tumor except :**
   A. Precocious puberty
   B. Acute abdomen
   C. Postmenopausal bleeding
   D. Hyperestrogenemia

234. **Staging of ca endometium with superficial myo- metrial involvement & size of uterine cavity 10 cms is :**
   A. Ia
   B. Ib
   C. IIa
   D. IIb

235. **Match List-I (Ovarian tumours) with List-II (Nature of neoplasm) and select the correct answer using the codes given below the Lists :**

List-I		List -II	
A. Dysgerminoma		1.	Highly malignant
B. Theca-Lutein cyst		2.	Chances of maligancy 50%
C. Serous cystadenoma		3.	Rare chance of malignancy
D. Dermoid cyst of the ovary		4.	Potentially malignant
		5.	Non-neoplastic cyst of the ovary

   Codes :

	a	b	c	d
a.	4	1	2	3
b.	2	4	3	5
c.	1	5	2	3
d.	1	5	3	2

236. **Simple cystic teratoma is seen in age group:**
   A. < 70 yrs
   B. 20 - 40 yrs
   C. 40 - 60 yrs
   D. 65 yrs

237. **Retention of urine is seen in the following type of cervical fibroid:**
   A. Anterior
   B. Posterior
   C. Central
   D. Lateral

Ans.	230. A	231. A	232. B	233. NONE	234. B
	235. B	236. C	237. B		

238. A female patient has adenocarcinoma uterus along with sarcoma of uterus is known as :
   A. Heterologous sarcoma
   B. Homologous sarcoma
   C. Sarcoma Uterus
   D. Mixed Mullerian carcinogenesis

239. Precursor lesions of invasive endometrial carcinoma include the following except :
   A. Cystic hyperplasia
   B. Adenomatons hyperplasia
   C. Atypical hyperplasia
   D. Carcinoma-in-situ
   E. Stump carcinoma

240. A patient is diagnosed to have CIN II. She approaches you for advice. You can definitely tell her the risk of lesion progressing to malignancy as :
   A. 5%   B. 15%
   C. 60%   D. 30%

241. Laparotomy of a lady with a suspected ovarian tumor showed bilaterally enlarged ovaries with smooth surfaces. Histology showed mucin secreting cells with a signet ring appearance. What is the likely diagnosis :
   A. Primary adenocarcinoma of ovary
   B. Granulosa cell tumor
   C. Krukenberg tumor
   D. Dysgerminoma

242. For females, untrue is :
   A. All adenexal masses in postmenopausal are malignant
   B. All adenexal masses above 8 cm are to be explored
   C. 75% of adenexal masses in perimenopausal females are benign
   D. If the patient is postmenopausal ovarian enlargement should be investigated promptly regardless of size

243. Schiller Duval bodies are seen in :
   A. Endodermal sinus tumor
   B. Granulosa cell tumor
   C. Choriocarcinoma
   D. Arrhenoblastoma

244. Consider the following malignant ovarian tumours :
   1. Disgerminoma
   2. Serous cystadenocarcinoma
   3. Malignant teratoma

Ans.	238. D	239. E	240. A	241. C	242. A	243. A
	244. D					

Which of these tumours are more common in children and adolescents as compared to older women ?

A. 1, 2 and 3   B. 1 and 2
C. 2 and 3   D. 1 and 3

245. A young patient is diagnosed to have choriocarcinoma. The treatment of choice is :

A. Hysterectomy
B. Chemotherapy
C. Chemotherapy followed by hysterectomy
D. Hysterectomy followed by chemotherapy

246. Vesicular mole in a 40 years old women is best treated by :

A. Total hysterctomy
B. Subtotal hysterectomy
C. Hysterotomy and ligation
D. Methotrexate therapy

247. A case of endometrial carcinoma stage II is best treated by :

A. Surgery
B. Preoperative radiotherapy followed by surgery
C. Prgestins followed by surgery
D. Chemothrapy followed by surgery

248. A 55 year old female presents with unilateral ovarian mass of 4" x 4". The correct management would be :

A. Call after 2 months and reassess
B. Give progesterone
C. Explore after admission
D. Emergency salpingo-oopherectomy

249. Treatment of choice in a 40 year old female with H. mole is :

A. Evacuation under anaesthesia
B. Partial hysterectomy
C. Total hysterectomy
D. Methotrexate

250. Intramural leiomyoma can cause all of the following except :

A. Antepartum haemorrhage
B. Post partum haemorrhage
C. Obstructed labour
D. Uterine inertia

251. Troploblast is formed by :

A. Chorion   B. Amnion
C. Yolk sac   D. None of the above

252. The serum tumor maker for trophoblastic tumor is :

A. α HCG   B. Calcitonin
C. β HCG   D. δ HCG

Ans.	245. B	246. A	247. C	248. C	249. C	250. A
	251. A	252. C				

253. Commonest site of metast
    A. Liver   B. Lung
    C. Brain   D. Cervical lymph nodes
254. Endometrial Hyperplasia is seen in :
    A. POCD
    B. Endometrial Ca.
    C. Sertoli leydig cell tumor
    D. Arrhenoblastoma
255. Drug of choice in choriocarcinoma :
    A. Methotrexate   B. 5 FU
    C. Vincristine   D. Procarbazine
256. Indication for methotrexate in a case of GTN is :
    A. Rising trend of HCG after evacuation
    B. Pretreatment HCG 200000 units
    C. Partial mole
    D. Rapid fall of HCg after evacuation
257. All of the following are prognostic factors in gestational trophoblastic
    disease [GTN] except :
    A. Number of childrn (living)
    B. Blood group
    C. HCG > 40000 IU
    D. Previous h/o molar pregnancy
258. A girl presents with primary amenorrhea; grade V thelarche, grade
    pubarache; no axillary hair; possible diagnosis :
    A. Testicular feminisation B. Mullerian agensis
    C. Turner's syndrome   D. Gonadal dysgenesis
259. Rekha, a 45 years woman with negative pap smear with postive
    endometrial curettage. Next managment will be :
    A. Radiation   B. Vaginal hysterectomy
    C. Conisation   D. Wetheim's hysterectomy
260. Most common ovarian tumor to undergo malignant change is :
    A. Serous cystadenoma   B. Mucinous cystadenoma
    C. Teratoma   D. Dermoid
261. 32 yr old para 2 pt has choreocarcinoma which is locali-sed to uterus,
    no metastasis, treatment is :
    A. Hysterectomy   B. Chemotherapy
    C. Combined   D. D & C
262. Adenocarcinoma of the uterus along with rhabdomyosarcoma of
    the uterus is seen, the condition is called :
    A. Homologous sarcoma

Ans.	253. B	254. B	255. A	256. A	257. A	258. A
	259. C	260. A	261. C	262. C		

B. Heterologous sarcoma

C. Mixed Mulleriam tumor

D. Carcinoma

263. **A 40 year old lady with CIN III. Best management is :**

A. Conisation

B. Wertheim's hysterectomy

C. Total abdominal hysterectomy

D. Punch biopsy

264. **Early blood metastases is seen in :**

A. Choriocarcinoma

B. Dysgerminoma

C. Serous carcinoma

D. Mucinous cystadenocarcinoma

265. **Most of the patients with ovarian malignancy present in which stage :**

A. I   B. II

C. III   D. IV

266. **A case of carcinoma cervix found to be in altered sensorium and with hiccups. Cause could be :**

A. Septicemia

B. Uremia

C. Erosion of blood vessels

D. Radiation nephritis

267. **A patient with carcinoma ovary involving both the ovaries had intact ovarian capsule and ascites with peritoneal washings positive for malignant cells. The stage of the patient is :**

A. Stage I   B. Stage 2

C. Stage 3   D. Stage 4

268. **A 12-year-old girl presented with a dysgermimoma cyst in the right ovary with intact capsule. The treatment of choice would be :**

A. Bilateral oophorectomy

B. Right oophorectomy

C. Right ovarian cystotomy

D. PAN hysterectomy

269. **HCG is not a marker for :**

A. Embryonal carcinoma

B. Endodermal sinus tumor

C. Polyembryoma

D. Dysgerminoma

Ans.	263. C	264. A	265. C	266. B	267.A	268. B
	269. B					

270. The following ovarian tumor is not benign :
    A. Teratoma   B. Dysgerminoma
    C. Brenner tumor   D. Fibroma

271. Commonest symptom of fallopian tube carcinoma :
    A. Profuse watery discharg
    B. Amenorrhoea
    C. Dysmenorrhoea
    D. Pain

272. Degeneration occuring in fibroid are all except :
    A. Haline   B. Cancerous
    C. Dystrophic   D. Red
    E. Cystic

273. Cyclical retention of urine is seen in :
    A. Subserous myoma
    B. Cervical fibroid
    C. Submucous myoma
    D. Fundal myoma

274. Young women whose mothers took diethylstibestrol during pregnancy are likely to develop one of the following genital malignancy:
    A. Squamous-cell carcinoma
    B. Adenosquamous carcinoma
    C. Papillary adenocarcinoma
    D. Clear-cell adenocarcinoma

275. A 45 yr old female is having bilateral ovarian mass, ascites and omental caking on CT Scan. There is high possibility that the patient is having :
    A. Benign Ovarian Tumor
    B. Malignant Epithelial Ovarian tumor
    C. Dysgerminoma of ovary
    D. Lymphoma of ovary

276. The worst prognosis in carcinoma endometrium is seen in which of the following types :
    A. Pappilary type   B. Adenocarcinoma
    C. Squamous type   D. Clear cell type

277. Consider the following :
    1. Cervix
    2. Breast
    3. Endometrium
    The risk of carcinoma of which of these is increased by   obesity :
    A. 1 and 2   B. 1 and 3
    C. 2 and 3   D. 1, 2 and 3

Ans.	270. B	271. A	272. E	273. B	274. D	275. B
	276. D	277. C				

278. **How much is the risk of ovarian cancer increased above normal in a woman with nonautosomal dominant genotype with one first degree relative with ovarian cancer?**

    A 2-3 times   B   5 times

    C 10 times.   D   20 times.

279. **What is the most common method for detecting early stage ovarian cancer?**

    A Evaluation of vague gastrointestinal symptoms.

    B Palpation of an asymptomatic mass during routine pelvic examination

    C Screening CA 125.

    D Screening vaginal ultrasound.

280. **Which ultrasound finding with an adnexal mass is most suspicious for**

    A. 8 cm. in diameter.

    B. Several internal excrescences.

    C. Cystic with two thin septations

    D. Free pelvic fluid

281. **Bluish suburethral nodule seen in lower 1/3rd of vagina is suggestive of:**

    A. Choriocarcinoma

    B. Carcinoma vagina

    C. Carcinoma cervix

    D. Carcinoma vulva

282. **Ca 125 is increased in the following conditions, except :**

    A. Endometriosis

    B. Dysgerminoma ovary

    C. Endometrioid carcinoma ovary

    D. Colorectal malignancy

283. **Primary neoplasm of retroperitoneal soft tissue is :**

    A. Seminoma   B. Teratoma

    C. Teratocaranoma   D. Chriocarcinoma

284. **Commonest cancer of vulva is :**

    A. Sq. cell type   B. Adenocarcinoma

    C. Columnar cell type   D. Transitional cell type

285. **Carcinoma vulva first spreads to ——— lymph nodes :**

    A. Iliac   B. Hypogastric

    C. Obturator   D. Inguinal

286. **Commonest tumor of female urethra is :**

    A. Transitional cell type   B. Adenocarcinoma

    C. Sq. cell type   D. Columnar cell type

Ans.	278. A	279. B	280. B	281. A	282. B	283. A
	284. A	285. D	286. C			

287. Commonest neoplasm of urogenital tract of infants and young children is :
A. Rhabdomysosarcoma B. Liposarcoma
C. Sq. cell type D. Transitional cell type

288. Commonest carcinoma of endometrium is :
A. Adenocarcinoma B. Adenocanthoma
C. Adenosquamous D. Sq. cell type

289. Carcinosarcoma may arise in :
A. Uterus B. Cervix
C. Vagina D. Ovary

290. The worst prognosis for Renal cell carcinoma is :
A. Vascular invasion
B. Associated with hypercalcemia
C. Presence of Hematuria
D. Size more than 5 cm

291. Primary germ cell tumors of the testis usually occur in young males with the exception of :
A. Embryonal carcinoma B. Spermatocytic seminoma
C. Polyembryoma D. Teratocarcinoma

292. Prognosis is best in which histologic type of renal carcinoma :
A. Pure clear cell type B. Granular cell type
C. Spindle cell type D. Mixed type

293. Following changes may occur in renal cell carcinoma except :
A. Increased leucocytic alk. phosphatase
B. Polycythemia
C. Hypercalcemia
D. Leucocytosis

294. Most reliable prognostic indicator of kidney and ureter excised for neoplasm of renal pelvis is :
A. Hematuria
B. Extension beyond renal parenchyma
C. Granular deposits
D. None

295. Hypernephroma :
A. Is a squamous cell carcinoma
B. Arises from the adrenals
C. Is yellow on cut section
D. Affects females predominantly

296. Commonest neoplasm of the urinary bladder is :
A. Squamous cell carcinoma

Ans.	287. A	288. A	289. A	290. A	291. B	292. A
	293. A	294. B	295. C	296. C		

B. Adenocarcinoma
C. Transitional cell carcinoma
D. Undifferentiated carcinoma
E. Sarcoma

297. Most of the testicular tumours arise from :
A. Leydig cells   B. Germ cells
C. Sertoli cells   D. Primitive gonadal stroma

298. Prognosis of Renal cell carcinoma is worst when :
A. Size more than 5 cm
B. Hematuria present
C. Vascular invasion is seen
D. Associated with hypercalcemia

299. Follicular ovarian cysts are seen in :
A. Tubal pregnancy   B. Molar pregnancy
C. Fibroid uterus   D. Threatened abortion

300. The most common type of malignancy of Renal pelvis is :
A. Squamous cell carcinoma
B. Transitional cell carcinoma
C. Adenocarcinoma
D. Mixed tumor

301. Nephroblastoma is most likely to occur at the age of :
A. 2 years   B. 20 years
C. 50 years   D. 70 years

302. Which is not true regarding renal cell carcinoma :
A. Arises from proximal convoluted tubules
B. More common in females
C. May associated with varicocele
D. May invade renal vein

303. Follicular ovarian cysts are seen in :
A. Molar pregnancy   B. Tubal pregnancy
C. Fibroid Uterus   D. Threatened abortion

304. All of the following are true of squamous metaplasia of the urinary bladder except :
A. Commonly associated with inflammatory disease
B. It is precancerous
C. Often occur within diverticulae of the bladder
D. Can occur in women on estrogen therapy

305. For Sq. cell Ca of bladder true is :
A. Dysplasia
B. Malignant trnasformation Metaplasia
C. Nitrosamine associated
D. Aniline dye

Ans.	297. B	298. C	299. B	300. B	301. A	302. B
	303. A	304. B	305. B			

306. Renal adenocarcinoma is caused by following except :
A. Cigarette
B. Cadmium
C. Balkan nephropathy
D. Von Hippel Londau disease

307. Krukenberg tumour of ovary arises form :
A. Breast   B. Stomach
C. Liver   D. Rectum

308. The following is the commonest tumour of urinary bladder :
A. Papilloma
B. Adenocarcinoma
C. Transitional cell carcinoma
D. Squamous cell carcinoma

309. All of the following predispose to carcinoma bladder except :
A. D-naphthylamine   B. Smoking
C. Schistosomiasis   D. Tuberculous cystitis

310. Urinary cytology is a useful screening test for   diagnosis of :
A. Renal cell carcinoma   B. Wilm's tumor
C. Urothelial carcinoma   D. Carcinoma prostate

311. The commonest side of metastasis of carcinoma prostate is :
A. Lungs   B. Liver
C. Bones   D. Brain

312. Best indication of testicular biopsy is :
A. Necrospermia   B. Pyospermia
C. Oligospermia   D. Azoospermia

313. People at risk for developing bladder cancer are following except :
A. Aniline dye factories worker
B. Rubber & cable industries
C. SS Auramine & magenta
D. Zinc & Aluminium

314. Most malignant tumor of the urinary bladder is histologically classified as :
A. Squamous cell carcinoma
B. Adeno carcinoma
C. Fibrosarcoma
D. Transitional cell carcinoma

315. Anaemia in Wilm's tumour is :
A. Microcytic hypochromic
B. Normocytic normochromic
C. Macrocytic
D. All of the above

Ans.	306. C	307. B	308. C	309. D	310. C	311. C
	312. D	313. D	314. D	315. B		

316. **The commonest testicular malignancy in children :**
    A. Infantile Embryonal carcinoma
    B. Chorio carcinoma
    C. Seminoma
    D. Teratoma

317. **The commonest tumour of renal pelvis and ureter is histologically:**
    A. Transitional cell type   B. Papillary cell type
    C. Squamous cell type   D. Adenocarcinoma

318. **Meig syndrome is most commonly seen with :**
    A. Fibroma
    B. Dysgerminoma
    C. Papillary cystadenocarcinoma
    D. Granulosa cell tumor

319. **The most common testicular tumor is :**
    A. Seminoma   B. Benign teratoma
    C. Malignant teratoma   D. Embryonal carcinoma

320. **Microscopic picture of seminoma testis :**
    A. Sheets of lymphocytes in homogneous background
    B. Glandular with papillary outgrowth
    C. Dermoid elements
    D. Hyperchromatic nuclei in eosinophilic cytoplasm

321. **All of the following are true of squamous metaplasia of the urinary bladder except :**
    A. Commonly associated with inflammatory disease
    B. It is precancerous
    C. Often occur within diverticulae of the   bladder
    D. Can occur in women on estrogen therapy

322. **The following testicular tumour has benign course :**
    A. Teratoma   B. Choriocarcinoma
    C. Seminoma   D. Leydig cell tumor

323. **Esthesio neuroblastoma would be found in :**
    A. Eustachian canal   B. Nasal cavity
    C. Mediastinum   D. Scrotum

324. **Dysgerminomas of the ovary are characterized by all of the following except :**
    A. Sheets of large polygonal or round cells with clear of light staining cytoplasm
    B. Fibrous storma infiltrated by lymphocytes
    C. Multinucleated foreign body giant cells
    D. Crystalloids of Reinke

Ans.	316. C	317. A	318. A	319. A	320. A	321. B
	322. B	323. B	324. D			

325. All of the following are germ cell tumours of testis except :
   A. Seminoma
   B. Sertoli cell tumour
   C. Teratom
   D. Mixed tumour
326. Metastasis from a renal cell carcinoma is commonly seen in all of the following except :
   A. Liver
   B. Spleen
   C. Lungs
   D. Bones
327. Seminoma is a counterpart of :
   A. Choriocarcinoma
   B. Dermoid
   C. Hilus cell tumou
   D. Dysgerminoma
328. Most common type of vaginal carcinoma is :
   A. Botryoid
   B. Squamous carcinoma
   C. Adenocarcinoma
   D. Melanoma
329. All are true of prostatic intra epithelial neoplasia (PIN) except :
   A. Overexpression of bcl-2 seen
   B. Intracinar proliferation
   C. Nuclear atypia
   D. > 50% show PCNA
330. Ovarian Ca associated with endometrial hyperplasia :
   A. Dysgerminoma
   B. Granulosa cell tumor
   C. Fibroma
   D. Mucinous cystadenoma
331. Wilm's tumor is best treated by :
   A. Surgery
   B. Radiotherapy
   C. (A) + (B)
   D. (A) + (B) + Chemotherapy
332. Anline, bilharzia, magenta and exfoliative cytology are related in terms of :
   A. Carcinoma of the colon
   B. Carcinoma of the cervix
   C. Bronchial tumours
   D. Bladder tumours
333. Haematuria at the begining of micturition is indicative of :
   A. Bladder neck pathology
   B. Renal pathology
   C. Benign prostatic hypertrop
   D. Urethral pathology
   E. None of the above
334. Earliest symptom of Wilm's tumour is :
   A. Hematuria
   B. Pyrexia
   C. Abdominal tumuor
   D. Metastaes

Ans.	325. B	326. B	327. D	328. B	329. A	330. B
	331. D	332. D	333. D	334. C		

335. **T2 stage Ca bladder is :**
   A. Mucosal invasion
   B. Submucosal invasion
   C. Muscularis mucosa involvment
   D. Pelvic tissue involvement

336. **Anaemia in Wilm tumour is :**
   A. Microcytic hypochromic
   B. Normocytic normochromic
   C. Macrocytic
   D. None of the above

337. **While giving, bath mother noticed an abdominal mass (unilateral) in 1.5 year old boy, the mass was not crossing midline and there was hemiatrophy . The diagonsis is :**
   A. Wilm's tumour
   B. Neuroblastoma
   C. Adenocarcinoma kidney
   D. Horse shoe kidney

338. **Most malignant renal tumuor is :**
   A. Grawitz tumor
   B. Paplillary tumors
   C. Squamous cell carcinoma of renal pelvis
   D. Wilm's tumor

339. **In surgery for pheochromocytoma, hypotension is because of :**
   A. Removal of catecholamines
   B. Resistance to catecholamines
   C. Endogenous substance
   D. Decreased blood volume

340. **Features of phaeochromocytoma include all except :**
   A. Pallor
   B. Hypoglycaemia
   C. Increased arterial tension
   D. Blurring of vision

341. **Features of vesical papilloma include all except :**
   A. Pain in perineum   B. Intemittent haematuria
   C. Painless haematuria   D. Clot retention

342. **In a clear cell carcinoma of the kidney with a solitary pulmonary metastasis, proceed with :**
   A. Symptomatic treatment
   B. Removal of the diseased kidney
   C. Chemotherapy
   D. Radiotherapy of lung and affected kidney

Ans.	335. C	336. B	337. A	338. C	339. A	340. B
	341. A	342. B				

343. **Wilm's tumour of the kidney :**
    A. Occurs predominantly in adults
    B. May have both adenomatous and carcinomatous segments
    C. Is radioresistant
    D. Is usually small
344. **Which of the following is most useful in distinguishing a renal carcinoma :**
    A. Intravenous urogram   B. Retrograde pyelogram
    C. Radio-active venogram   D. Renal arteriogram
345. **Medical adrenalectomy in recurrent carcinoma breast is done with:**
    A. Steroids   B. Aminoglutethimide
    C. Tamoxifen   D. Radiotherapy
346. **The following testicular tumour has a benign course :**
    A. Teratoma   B. Choriocarcinoma
    C. Seminoma   D. Leydig cell tumour
347. **Recognised clinical features of Wilm's tumour include each of the following except :**
    A. Distant metastasis in lungs
    B. Silent renal mass
    C. Stripped calcification in tumour mass
    D. Distortion of renal pelvis on IVP
348. **The following procedure is not useful in the diagnosis of phaeochromocytomas :**
    A. Phentolamine test   B. Histamine test
    C. Glucagon infusion   D. Urinary catecholamines
349. **An 82 years old man underwent open prostatectomy. Histology revealed benign nodular hyperplasia with an area of focal adenocarcinoma and following further treatment recommended :**
    A. Deep X-ray therapy   B. Stilboestrol therapy
    C. No treatment   D. Orchidectomy
350. **In phaeochromocytoma, treatment is by :**
    A. Beta blocker folowed by alpha blocker
    B. Alpha followed by beta blocker
    C. Both given together and later on alpha blocker
    D. Both given together and later on beta blocker
351. **Commonest type of cancer renal pelvis and upper ureter is :**
    A. Transitional cell carcinoma
    B. Adenocarcinoma
    C. Nephroblastoma
    D. Squamous cell carcinoma

Ans.	343. B	344. D	345. B	346. D	347. C	348. B
	349. C	350. A	351. A			

352. **Which does not occur in Adrenal cortical tumors :**
    A. Striae over body   B. DM
    C. ↑ACTH   D. Hyperkalemia

353. Commonest symptom of pheochromocytoma is :
    A. Palpitation   B. Headache
    C. Sweating   D. Dyspnoea

354. **In hypernephroma, all are true except :**
    A. Usually adenocarcinoma
    B. It is radiosensitive
    C. Present with rapidly developing varicocele
    D. It arises from cortex, possibly from preexisting adenoma

355. **All are true about renal cell carcinoma except :**
    A. Arises from PCT   B. Invades renal vein
    C. More common in femal D. Hematuria may occur

356. **Epidermoid carcinoma of renal pelvis is usually associated with :**
    A. Multiple papillomas   B. Pelvic calculus
    C. TB kidney   D. Filariasis

357. **Malignancy and phaeochromocytoma is diagnosed by :**
    A. Vascular invasion
    B. Anaplasia
    C. Increase in nuclear cytoplasmic ratio
    D. All of the above

358. **Regarding angiohematomas of kidney which is   incorrect :**
    A. Presents with hypertension
    B. Loin pain
    C. Nephrectomy is the treatment of choice
    D. Bleeding is self limited

359. **All are true regarding Wilm's tumor except :**
    A. Good prognosis in infants
    B. Pre operative use of Actinomycin D
    C. Post operative radiotherapy
    D. Neuroblastoma is the commonest differential diagnosis

360. **The commonest tumour of urinary bladder is :**
    A. Papilloma
    B. Adenocarcinoma
    C. Transitional cell carcinoma
    D. Squamous cell carcinoma

Ans.	352. C	353. B	354. B	355. C	356. B	357. A
	358. C	359. B	360. C			

361. Duke's Stage C2 refers to carcinoma :
    A. Bladder penetrating the extravesical fat
    B. Bladder with metastasis to internal iliac lymph nodes
    C. With histological features of 75% anaplastic cells
    D. Rectum with metastasis to inferior mesenteric lymph nodes

362. One of the following is not a common adrenal gland tumour?
    A. Haemangioma   B. Myelolipoma
    C. Aldosteronoma   D. Phaeochromocytoma

363. Symptoms of Wilm's tumur include all except :
    A. Haematuria   B. Dysuria
    C. Pyrexia   D. Mass abdomen

364. In neuroblastoma, the following are raised except :
    A. MHPG   B. VMA
    C. HVA   D. None of the above

365. The following may be the presentation of Grawitz's tumour except :
    A. Polycythemia   B. Nephrotic syndrome
    C. Hypertension   D. Phaeochromocytoma

366. The least common site of metastasis of Wilm's tumour is :
    A. Liver   B. Lungs
    C. Bones   D. Brain

367. The following drugs may be useful in the treatment of Wilm's tumour except :
    A. Actinomycin D   B. Vincristine
    C. Cyclophosphamide   D. 5-FU

368. The irradiation of the Wilm's tumour is recommended in the following situations except :
    A. Preoperatively
    B. Postoperatively
    C. Alongwith chemotherapy
    D. Postoperatively alongwith chemotherapy

369. In Wilm's tumour, X-ray of abdomen characteristically shows —
    — type of calcification :
    A. Speckled   B. Diffuse
    C. Corvilinear   D. Any of the above

370. Treatment of choice for adenocarcinoma of kidney is :
    A. Surgery   B. Radiotherapy
    C. Chemotherapy   D. Immunotherapy

371. True about phaeochromocytoma is :
    A. Is a soft blue coloured malignant tumor
    B. Presents as yellowish discolouration of face

Ans.	361. D	362. A	363. B	364. A	365. D	366. D
	367. D	368. A	369. C	370. A	371. B	

    C. Urinary HIAA levels are increased

    D. Hypertension is always paraoxysmal

372. **Treatment of Papillary tumor of base of bladder is :**

    A. TUR   B. Cystodiathermy

    C. Bladder removal   D. Radiotherapy

373. **Consider the following conditions :**

    1. Hydronephrosis

    2. Wilm's tumour

    3. Neuroblastoma

    4. Pheochromocytoma

    5. Tumour in undescended testis

    The common abdominal lumps in children are due to :

    A. 1,2,3   B. 1,4,5

    C. 2,3,4   D. 1,2,5

374. **In pheochromocytoma there is increased level of :**

    A. Serum HMA   B. Serum bradykinin

    C. Urinary VMA   D. All of the above

375. **Agent of choice for intravesical therapy for carcinoma in situ of bladder cancer following endoscopic treatment is?**

    A. BCG   B. Mitomycin C

    C. Adriamycin   D. Thiotepa

376. **The commonest mode of spread of carcinoma prostate is :**

    A. Lymphatics   B. Blood vessels

    C. Direct   D. None of the above

377. **Regarding treatment of prostatic cancer which is incorrect ?**

    A. Radical prostatectomy has great value

    B. Treatment with oestrogens plays great role

    C. Orchidectomy has a role

    D. Supravoltage X-ray therapy is sometimes used

378. **In testicular Ca, investigation not done is :**

    A. Aortography   B. CT scan

    C. Biopsy   D. Serum AF

379. **The most common site for carcinoma of the prostate :**

    A. Anterior lobe   B. Posterior lobe

    C. Median lobe   D. Right lateral lobe

380. **Commonest testicular malignancy is :**

    A. Seminoma   B. Teratoma

    C. Choriocarcinoma   D. Embryonal cell carcinoma

Ans.	372. B	373. A	374. D	375. A	376. B	377. A
	378. C	379. B	380. A			

381. 80 year old man underwent transurethral prostatectomy biopsy and revealed foci of adenocarcinoma. Next line of management :
A. Radiotherapy   B. Hormonal therapy
C. Surgery   D. No further treatment

382. Testicular tumour with cartilage elements is:
A. Seminoma
B. Teratoma
C. Embryonal cell tumour
D. Interstitial cell tumor

383. The most common testicular tumor of childhood is :
A. Interstitial cell tumor   B. Teratoma
C. Seminoma   D. Chorio carcinoma

384. Osteoblastic secondaries in bone are seen with :
A. Ca breast   B. Ca. stomach
C. Ca. prostate   D. All of the above

385. Testicular malignancy commonest in underscended testes is :
A. Seminoma   B. Teratoma
C. Embryonal cell Ca   D. Mixed

386. Which of the following testicular tumours is the most radiosensitive ?
A. Teratoma   B. Embryoma
C. Terato-carcinoma   D. Seminoma
E. Chorio-carcinoma

387. Prostatic cancer metastasizes most frequently to :
A. Spine   B. Femur
C. Lung   D. Rectum
E. Liver

388. Which is true regarding seminoma testis :
A. Occurs in undescerded testis
B. Is radioresistant
C. Occurs in a relatively younger age group
D. Is highly malignant

389. In tumour testis is suspected which test is done :
A. Tapping the hydrocele and doing pathological examination of fluid
B. Exploration and removal of testis
C. Needle biopsy
D. None of the above

390. Carcinoma prostate is associated with :Karnataka 1993
A. Increased serum alkaline phosphatase
B. Osteosclerotic secondaries

Ans.	381. D	382. B	383. B	384. C	385. A	386. D
	387. A	388. A	389. A	390. B		

    C. Obturator lymphadenopathy

    D. All of the above

391. **Tumor marker for testicular teratoma is :**

    A. Beta HCG   B. Testosteoine

    C. LDH   D. LH

392. ↑ **HCG titres are diagnostic of :**

    A. Hepatic cell carcinoma B. Colonic carcinoma

    C. Trophoblastic tumour D. Seminoma testis

393. **Definite precancerous condition of penis include all except :**

    A. Leukoplakia of glans

    B. Penile papilloma

    C. Chronic balanoprosthitis

    D. Paget's disease of the penis

394. **Each of the following features is characteristic of extragonadal teratomas except :**

    A. Midline location   B. Multiplicity of tissues

    C. Origin from germ cells D. Radiosensitivity

395. **Following are the germinal variety of Testicular Neoplasms except :**

    A. Seminoma

    B. Yolk sac tumour

    C. Leydig cell tumour

    D. Endodermal sinus tumour

396. **Malignant changes of testis occurs in :**

    A. Crypto-orchidism   B. Trauma

    C. Hydrocele   D. Pyocele

397. **Man aged 60 has testicular tumor; most likely to be :**

    A. Germ cell   B. Sertoli cell

    C. Teratocarcinoma   D. Lymphoma

398. **Commonest bone involved in carcinoma prostate is :**

    A. Spine   B. Rips

    C. Pelvis   D. Femur

399. **A patient suspected to have prostatic carcinoma. The best investigation to evaluate him would be :**

    A. TRUS   B. Expressed prostatic secretions

    C. CT scan   D. MRI

400. **Treatment of choice of stage I seminoma is :**

    A. High inguinal orchidectomy with radiotherapy

    B. Intravenous chemotherapy

    C. Trans-scrotal orchidectomy

    D. High inguinal orchidectomy

Ans.	391. A	392. C	393. C	394. D	395. C	396. A
	397. D	398. C	399. A	400. A		

401. Most specific tumor marker for prostate is :
    A. Acid phosphatase
    B. Alkaline phospohatase
    C. Prostate specific antig
    D. HCG

402. Mcknow's operation is done for which carcinoma?
    A. Carcinoma oesophagus
    B. Ca stomach
    C. Bronchogenic carcinoma
    D. Ca. colon

403. Eight year old boy presented with swelling in left eye of 3 months duration. Examination revealed proptosis of left eye with preserved vision. Right eye is normal. CT Scan revealed intraorbital extra conal mass lesion. Biopsy revealed embryonal rhabdomyosarcoma. Metastatic work up was normal. The standard line of treatment is :
    A. Chemotherapy only
    B. Wide local excision
    C. Enucleation
    D. Chemotherapy and Radiation therapy

404. Radiation exposure during infancy has been linked to which one of the following carcinoma :
    A. Breast   B. Melanoma
    C. Thyroid   D. Lung

405. Increased expression of erb2 gene is associated with ?
    A. Breast cancer   B. Hodgkin's lymphoma
    C. NHL   D. Ca colon

406. CEA is elevated in which of the following malignancies ?
    A. Lung breast testis   B. Lung colon pancreas
    C. Breast colon testis D. Thyroid breast lung

407. Persistent nephrogram is seen in :
    A. Ureteric obstruction   B. Horseshoe kidney
    C. Renal tumour   D. Hydronephrosis

408. All the following are true about angiomyolipomas of kidneys except :
    A. Ultrasound is the investigation of choice
    B. It is associated with tuberous sclerosis
    C. It is considered a hamartoma
    D. It may present with flank pain
    E. Angiography may reveal aneurysms

Ans.	401. C	402. A	403. D	404. C	405. A	406. B
	407. C	408. A				

409. **Testicular tumors occur frequently in :**
     A. Testis with scrotal hernia
     B. Underscended abdominal testis
     C. Mumbs orchitis
     D. Following injury to testis

410. **All are related to development of bladder cancer except :**
     A. Tuberculosis   B. Bilharziasis
     C. Aniline dyes   D. Chronic irritation

NERVOUS SYSTEM

1. **Cronipharyngiomas have all the following features except :**
   A. They are encapuslated and firmly adherent to surrounding tissue
   B. They are usually cystic
   C. They form cords of stratified squamous epithelium
   D. They show frequent mitosis and pleomorphism

2. **Rarest form of posterior fossa tumor is :**
   A. Oligodendroglioma   B. Astrocytoma
   C. Ependymoma   D. Medullblastoma

3. **Nasopharangeal angiofibromas are most frequently seen in decade:**
   A. Second   B. Third
   C. Fourth   D. Fifth and sixth

4. **The following may be seen on histological examination of meningiomas except :**
   A. Melanin   B. Bone formation
   C. Xanthomatous change D. Mucin production

5. **The coomonest cause of intracranial metastasis is malignancy of :**
   A. Breast   B. Lungs
   C. Stomach   D. Testes

6. **The commonest supratentorial brain tumour in adults is :**
   A. Meningioma   B. Glioma
   C. Medulloblastoma   D. Craniopharyingioma

7. **Albumino-cytologic dissociation occurs in cases of :**
   A. Guillain Barre syndrome
   B. TBM
   C. Motor neurone disease
   D. Demyelinating disorder
   E. Any of the above

8. **The commonest supratentoiral tumour is :**
   A. Meningioma   B. Chordoma
   C. Glioma   D. Craniopharyngioma

9. **Commonest intracranial neoplasm is :**
   A. Fibroma   B. Glioma
   C. Meningioma   D. Medulloblastoma

Ans.	1. D	2. A	3. A	4. D	5. B	6. B
	7. A	8. C	9. B			

10. Brain scan showing a mass in the right cerebral hemisphere with calcification is :
   A. Oligodendroglioma   B. Astrocytoma
   C. Metastatic carcinoma   D. Brown tumour

11. Commonest type of intracranial tumour is :
   A. Astrocytoma   B. Medulloblatoma
   C. Meningioma   D. Neurofibroma
   E. Secondaries

12. Metastatic carcinoma is the most common form of malignant brain tumour in :
   A. Children under 10 years old
   B. Adults without a known primary tumor
   C. Children between 10 and 20 year old
   D. Adults with a known primary tumor

13. Glioblastoma multiforme may occur in the following except :
   A. Cerebrum of adult
   B. Cerebellum of child
   C. Spinal cord of adult
   D. Adrenal medulla of child

14. All the following are true about primary CNS lymphoma except :
   A. Most common type is diffuse histiocytic type
   B. Most are of T-cell origin
   C. Multicentric location
   D. Causes focal signs

15. Commonest primary brain tumour is:
   A. Astrocytoma   B. Glioblastoma
   C. Ependymoma   D. Meningioma

16. Commonest intramedullary spinal tumour is:
   A. Chordoma   B. Meningioma
   C. Ependymoma   D. Oligodendroglioma

17. The most common site of chondroma in vertebral column is:
   A. Sacro-coccygeal   B. Cervico-Thoracic
   C. Thoracic   D. Thoraco lumber

18. In children,intracranial tumours are more common in:
   A. Anterior fossa
   B. Middle fossa
   C. Posterior fossa
   D. Equal incidences in all fossa

19. The commonest of triad of brain SOL are all except :
   A. Headache   B. Vomiting
   C. Diplopia   D. Papilloedema

Ans.	10. A	11. E	12. D	13. B	14. B	15. A
	16. C	17. C	18. C	19. C		

20. **Empty sella syndrome is often characterized by:**
    A. Pituitary tumour   B. Cretinism
    C. Acromegaly   D. None of the above

21. **Which of the following lesions of the thymus is most commonly associated with myasthenia gravis?**
    A. Lymphoepthelioma
    B. Teratoma
    C. Granulomatous thymoma
    D. None of the above

22. **The following are true about the characterisitics of sacrococcygeal teratoma except :**
    A. One of the most common large tumours seen during first three months of life
    B. Males are more often affected than females
    C. Tumours arise between sacrum and rectum
    D. Prone to become malignant

23. **Non metastatic neurological manifestation in bronchogenic carcinoma includes all the following, except :**
    A. Cerebellar degeneration   B. Hoarseness of voice
    C. Myopathy   D. Peripheral neuropathy

24. **The commonest supratentorial tumour in adults is:**
    A. Meningioma   B. Glioma
    C. Medulloblastoma   D. Craniopharyngioma

25. **Which of the following is a cystic cranial tumour :**
    A. Craniopharyngioma   B. Astrocytoma
    C. Medulloblastoma   D. Ependynoma

26. **True about meningioma is all except :**
    A. 19% of brain tumour
    B. Parasagittal meningioma common
    C. Reactive hyperostosis
    D. Flat
    E. Arises from meninges

27. **Malignant astrocytoma is most common in:**
    A. Frontal lobe   B. Temporal lobe
    C. Parietal lobe   D. Cerebellum

28. **Patient presents with high fever, signs of raised ICT and a past history of chronic otitis media. Likely diagnosis :**
    A. Brain abscess
    B. Pyogenic meningitis
    C. Acute subarachnoid haemorrhage
    D. Acute osteomyelitis of skull bone

Ans.	20. D	21. A	22. B	23. B	24. B	25. A
	26. D	27. A	28. B			

29. **Dumbell tumour is seen in:**
A. Meningioma   B. Neurofibroma
C. Epidendymoma   D. Thymoma

30. **A-10 year old child presents with midline cerebellar tumour. Most likely diagnosis is :**
A. Medulloblastoma   B. Astrocytoma
C. Glioblastoma   D. Hemangioblastoma

31. **The most malignant brain tumour is:**
A. Glioblastoma multiforme
B. Spongioblastoma
C. Ependymoma
D. Oligodendroglioma

32. **A brain tumour which has CSF metastasis and is radiosensitive:**
A. Ependymoma   B. Medulloblastoma
C. Pinealoblastoma   D. Astrocytoma

33. **Metastasis outside the brain occurs in brain tumour:**
A. Crainopharyngioma   B. Glioblastoma
C. Medulloblastoma   D. Hemangioblastoma

34. **The most common tumour of pineal gland is:**
A. Lipoma   B. Astrocytoma
C. Haemangioma   D. Germinoma

35. **Most common endocrine tumor of pituitary is :**
A. GH Tumor   B. ACTH tumor
C. Prolactinoma   D. TSH secreting tumor

36. **Among following, CNS tumor with best prognosis is :**
A. Cerebral astrocytoma B. Cerebellar astrocytoma
C. Medulloblastoma   D. Glioblastoma

37. **Pituitary tumor produces :**
A. Bitemporal hemianopia
B. Binasal hemianopia
C. Unilateral quadrantopia
D. Increase in blind spot only

38. **Blood brain barrier is not present in following except :**
A. Neurohypophysis   B. Area postrema
C. Subfornical organ   D. IV ventricle

39. **Stereolactic radiosurgery is done for :**
A. Glioblastoma multiforme
B. Medullo blastoma spinal cord
C. Opendyomoma
D. AV malformation of brain

Ans.	29. B	30. A	31. A	32. B	33. C	34. D
	35. C	36. C	37. C	38. D	39. A	

40. Suprasellar calcification is seen in following except :
    A. Craniopharyngioma   B. Meningioma
    C. Calcified pineal gland D. Pituitary adenoma
41. 'Bare Orbit' appearance of skull is seen in :
    A. Multiple myeloma   B. Meningioma
    C. Neurofibromatosis   D. Craniopharyngioma
42. Commonest calcified brain tumour is :
    A. Craniopharyngioma   B. Meningioma
    C. Tuberculoma   D. Medulloblastoma
43. Intracranial calcification is seen in all except:
    A. Lipoma of corpus collosum
    B. Medulloblastoma
    C. Tuberculoma
    D. Ependymoma
    E. Neurofibromatosis
44. Which of the following brain tumors does not spread via CSF?
    A. Germ cell tumors   B. Medulloblastoma
    C. CNS Lymphoma   D. Craniopharyngioma

Ans.	40. D	41. C	42. A	43. B	44. D

HAEMATOLOGY

1. **Acute leukaemia may be caused by exposure to :**
   A. Benzene
   B. Vinyl chloride
   C. Nickel
   D. Naphthylamine

2. **Chromosomal abnormality seen in promyelocytic leukaemia :**
   A. 17-15t
   B. 21-9t
   C. 22-9t
   D. None

3. **Bone marrow infilteration is seen with the following except :**
   A. Retino blastoma
   B. Neuroblastoma
   C. Non-Hodgkin's lymphoma
   D. Wilm's tumour

4. **Triad of gross hematuria, pain and abdominal mass in renal cell carcinoma is present in :**
   A. 10%
   B. 30%
   C. 40%
   D. 60%

5. **CML is characterised by all except :**
   A. Leukocytosis
   B. Thrombocytosis
   C. Increaed leukocyte alkaline phosphatase
   D. Increased serum vitamin B12

6. **Which of the following statements about acute lymphoblastic leukaemia (ALL) is true ?**
   A. B-cell ALL has the best prognosis
   B. Girls are more often affected than boys
   C. Stained blood films commonly show Auer rods
   D. Widespread lymph node enlargement may occur

7. **Acute myelogenous leukemia is cytochemically :**
   A. Peroxidase negative
   B. ANE positive
   C. NCE positive
   D. Sudan Black B negative

8. **Commonest leukemia in bone is :**
   A. CML
   B. CLL
   C. ALL
   D. AML

9. **The commonest leukaemia inNorthern India is :**
   A. AML
   B. CML
   C. ALL
   D. CLL

Ans.	1. A	2. A	3. C	4. A	5. C	6. D
	7. C	8. A	9. B			

10. **All are seen in multiple myeloma except :**
    A. Plasmacytosis>2% on bone marrow
    B. Lytic bone lesion
    C. Hypercalcemia
    D. Serum alk. phosphatase activity

11. **In multiple myeloma, best indicator of prognosis is :**
    A. Serum β2-microglobulins
    B. No. of plasma cells in marrow
    C. Level of Ca++
    D. None of the above

12. **Hairy cell leukemia affects :**
    A. T. cell   B. B. cell
    C. Macrophage   D. Monocyte

13. **Philadelphia chromosome (Ph1) is commonly associated with :**
    A. Chronic lymphatic leukemia
    B. Leukemoid reaction
    C. Acute monocytic leukemia
    D. None of the above

14. **In multiple myeloma which of the following is not correct for diagnosis :**
    A. Plasmacytosis   B. G-spike
    C. Lytic lesion   D. Normal Alk PO4

15. **Type of Leukaemia often associated with disseminated intravascular coagulation (DIC) :**
    A. L3   B. M2
    C. M3   D. M4

16. **Benign and malignant paraproteinemia is differentiated by :**
    A. Serum total protein
    B. Serum immunoglobulin
    C. Serum cryoglobulin
    D. Monoclonal light chain in urine

17. **Lacunar cells are seen in which type of Hodgkin's lymphoma :**
    A. Lymphocyte predominance
    B. Lymphocyte depletion
    C. Nodular sclerosing
    D. Mixed cellularity

18. **Mylopthisic anaemia is most commonly seen in:**
    A. Hodgkins lymphoma   B. Multiple myeloma
    C. Metastatic carcinoma D. Leukemia

Ans.	10. A	11. A	12. B	13. D	14. B	15. C
	16. B	17. C	18. D			

19.   LAP (Leucocyte alkaline phosphate) is increased in   all except :
A. CML   B.   ALL
C. PNH   D.   Leukemoid reaction

20.   Acute promyelocytic leukaemia (AML-M3) includes which of the following subtypes ?
A. Hypergranular and hypogranular type
B. Hypergranular and hypersegmented
C. Hypergranular and microgranular type
D. Hypogranular and microgranular type
E. Hypogranular and inclusion type

21.   Tumor associated with polycythemia vera :
A. Sarcoma
B   Cerebral haemangioma
C. Cerebelllar haemangioblastoma
D. Sturge Weber syndrome

22.   Increase in Alkaline phosphatase is seen in :
A. CML   B.   Leukemoid reaction
C. Eosinophilia   D.   Malaria

23.   CD-10 is seen in :
A. ALL   B.   CLL
C. HCL   D.   CML

24.   All of the following are poor prognostic factors for acute myeloid leukemias, except :
A. Age more than 60 yrs
B. Leucocyte count more than 1,00,000/microL
C. Secondary Leukemias
D. Presence of t(8-21)

25.   All of the following statements about Hairy cell leukemia are true except?
A. Splenomegaly is conspicuous
B. Results from an expansion of neoplastic T lymphocytes
C. Cells are positive for Tartarate Resistant Acid Phosphatase (TRAP)
D. The cells express CD25 consistently

Ans.	19. A	20. C	21. C	22. B	23. A	24. D
	25. B					

OSTEOLOGY

1. The usual site of glomus tumour is :
   A. Vertebrae   B. Skull
   C. Pelvis   D. Phalanges
2. Which of the following is characteristic histological finding in a case of chondroblastoma ?
   A. Osteoid formation
   B. Chondroid material with lacy calcification surrounding the chondroblasts
   C. Mucoid degeneration
   D. Presence of fibrous tissue and cartilage
3. Osteogenic sarcoma metastasizes to :
   A. Liver   B. Lung
   C. Brain   D. Regional lymphnodes
4. An osteoclastoma may resemble :
   A. Osteitis fibrocystica   B. Chondrosarcoma
   C. Osteosarcoma   D. None of the above
5. The common mode of presentation of a case of solitary bone cyst is :
   A. Pain
   B. Fracture
   C. Inflammation
   D. Expansion of the involved area
6. Giant cell tumour of bone is radiologically characterised by :
   A. Expansible osteolytic lesion
   B. Periosteal new bone formation as sun rays
   C. Onion peel appearance
   D. Stippled osteoporosis
7. Osteogenic sarcoma is more commonly found in the :
   A. Metaphyseal areas of long bones
   B. Diaphyseal areas of long bones
   C. Flat bones
   D. Epiphysis of long bones
8. A giant cell tumour histologically resemble :
   A. Aneurysmal bone cyst   B. Solitary bone cyst
   C. Chondroblastoma   D. None ossifying fibroma
   E. All the above

Ans.	1. D	2. B	3. B	4. A	5. B	6. A
	7. A	8. E				

9. **Bone tumour not seen in a child is :**
    A. Osteosarcoma   B. Osteoclastoma
    C. Chondrosarcoma   D. Multiple myeloma

10. **A lusterless black lesion under the great toe nail of a 50 years old patient, noticed for three months, is most likely to be :**
    A. Sub-ungual haematoma B. Malignant melanoma
    C. Chronic paronychia   D. Glomus tumour

11. **In a young female, common lower femur epiphyseal growth is :**
    A. Bone cyst   B. Giant cell tumor
    C. Ewing's tumor   D. Osteosarcoma

12. **The tumours that metastasize most readily to be are carcinomas of all of the following, except :**
    A. Thyroid   B. Breast
    C. Kidney   D. Rectum

13. **Ewing's tumour is :**
    A. Radio sensitive   B. Radioresistant
    C. Radiorecurrent   D. Radiocurable

14. **Tumours of bones and joints include following except :**
    A. Krukenberg tumour   B. Ameloblastoma
    C. Chrodoma   D. Synovioma
    E. Glomus tumour

15. **Destruction of the bone with the surrounding dense bone in :**
    A. Osteosarcoma   B. Fibrosarcoma
    C. Chondrosarcom   D. Ewing's tumour

16. **Aneurysmal bone cysts :**
    A. Are true aneurysms of nutrient arteries
    B. Occur only in flat bones
    C. Are the same is osseous haemangiomas
    D. Manifest as osteolytic lesions in long bones

17. **Osteogenic sarcoma develops in Paget's disease in —— patients :**
    A. 1%   B. 5%
    C. 15%   D. None

18. **Sclerotic metastatic lesions are found in case of :**
    A. Carcinoma stomach   B. Carcinoma lungs
    C. Carcinoma prostate   D. Carcinomas uterus
    E. Carcinoma oesophagus

19. **The most common site of origin of an osteoma is :**
    A. Spine   B. Pelvis
    C. Skull   D. Scapula
    E. Diaphysis of long bones

Ans.	9. D	10. B	11. B	12. D	13. A	14. A
	15. D	16. A	17. A	18. C	19. E	

20. **Codman's triangle :**
    A. is seen only in malignancies of bone
    B. is triangular, punched out area within the bone
    C. Is due to lifting up of peristeum
    D. Does not contain tumour tissue itself

21. **A 12-year old boy fell down and suffered acute pain in the should**
    Examintion revealed tenderness and swelling over the upper third
    humerus. X-ray revealed a pathological fracture through a transl
    cent area in the metaphysis with the bone expanded in fusiform ma
    ner with thin cortex and no periosteal reaction. The radiolucent ar
    extended up to the epiphyseal plate. The most likely diagnosis is :
    A. Ewing's sarcoma   B. Solitary bone cyst
    C. Giant cell tumour   D. Fibrous dysplasia

22. **An osteoblastoma histologically resemble closely to :**
    A. Osteoid osteoma   B. Osteosarcoma
    C. Osteoclastoma   D. Chondrosarcoma

23. **The following conditions has/have worst prognosis :**
    A. Primary chondrosarcoma
    B. Secondary sarcomatous changes in multiple chondromatosis
    C. Both
    D. None

24. **The most common tumour that involves bone is :**
    A. Giant cell tumour
    B. Chondrosarcoma
    C. Multiple myeloma
    D. Metastatic tumour from extraosseous sit

25. **The fate of untreated osteoid osteoma is :**
    A. Malignant malformation   B. Spontaneous healing
    C. Gradual healing   D. Remains as such

26. **Commonest benign tumour under 21 yrs of age :**
    A. Aneurysmal bone cyst   B. Osteochondroma
    C. Giant cell tumour   D. Osteoid osteoma

27. **Bone tumour metastatising to bone is :**
    A. Giant cell tumour   B. Ewing's sarcoma
    C. Chondro sarcoma   D. Osteosarcoma

28. **Tumor not arising from cartilage is :**
    A. Enchondroma   B. Osteoblastoma
    C. Chondrosarcoma   D. Osteochondroma

29. **Which of the following is a true neoplasm?**
    A. Osteoid osteoma   B. Osteochondroma
    C. Fibrosarcoma of bone   D. None of the above

Ans.	20. C	21. B	22. A	23. A	24. D	25. C
	26. B	27. B	28. B	29. A		

30. **Ivory osteoma commonly arises in the :**
A. Skull
B. Ribs
C. Pelvis
D. Vertebra

31. **Which of the following may present as solitary bone cyst ?**
A. Eosinophilic granuloma
B. Enchondroma
C. Giant cell tumour
D. Any of the above

32. **Radiologically, a chondromyxoid fibroma may closely resemble :**
A. Fibrous dysplasia
B. Chondrosarcoma
C. Non-osteogenic fibroma
D. None of the above

33. **The soft tissue sarcoma that invades bone is most often a :**
A. Synovioma
B. Angiosarcoma
C. Lipoarcoma
D. None of the above

34. **Osteoid osteoma has its site of origin in :**
A. The bone cortex
B. The periosteum
C. The medullary cavity
D. Any of the above

35. **Retinaculum cell sarcoma is considered a member of the :**
A. Osteogenic tumors
B. Metastatic tumours
C. Angiomatous tumors
D. Lymphoma

36. **Ewing's sarcoma can be confused histologically with :**
A. Osteosarcoma
B. Giant cell tumour
C. Myeloma
D. Osteomyelitis

37. **Treatment of choice of a confirmed giant cell tumour is :**
A. Deep X-ray therapy
B. Curettage and bone grafting
C. Resection of tumour bearing position of bone
D. Amputation

38. **Osseous haemangiomas usually occur in :**
A. Small bones
B. Long bones
C. Flat bones
D. Vertebrae

39. **Which of the following is rare (uncommon) site for secondaries ?**
A. Vertebrae
B. Skull
C. Pelvis
D. Forearm and leg bones

40. **Rossette formation (Histologically) is seen in fracture of :**
A. Chondroma
B. Chondrosarcoma
C. Neuroblastoma
D. Reticulum cell sarcoma

41. **Radiologically, a glomus tumour of bone resembles :**
A. Echondroma
B. Osteoid osteoma
C. Fibrous dysplasia
D. Paget's disease

Ans.	30. A	31. D	32. C	33. A	34. D	35. D
	36. D	37. C	38. D	39. D	40. C	41. A

42. Commonest site of chondroblastoma is :
    A. Epiphysis
    B. Diaphysis
    C. Metaphysis
    D. Soft tissues
    E. Periosteum
43. Osteoid osteoma is most commonly found in the age group of :
    A. 1-10 years
    B. 10-25 years
    C. 25-50 years
    D. Over 50 years
44. Soap bubble appearance is seen in:
    A. Osteolastoma
    B. Osteosarcoma
    C. Ewing's sarcoma
    D. Lymphom
45. In which of the following condition involving extre-mity, is excision of regional lymph nodes done :
    A. Osteoclastoma
    B. Synoval cell sarcoma
    C. Ewing's sarcoma
    D. Adamantioma
46. Bone cyst commonly occur in :
    A. Humerus
    B. Femur
    C. Tibia
    D. Spine
47. Which tumour does not arise from cartilage ?
    A. Enchondroma
    B. Osteochondroma
    C. Chondrosarcoma
    D. Osteoblastoma
48. An adolescent with lower femur swelling, calcified lung opacity with pneumothorax, most likely diagnosis is :
    A. Osteogenic sarcoma
    B. Osteoclastoma
    C. Ewings sarcoma
    D. Metastasis
49. The most common site of aneurysmal bone cyst is :
    A. Upper end of tibia
    B. Lower end of Humerus
    C. Pelvic bones
    D. Radius
50. Of the following, which is not a benign tumor?
    A. Chondroma
    B. Chordoma
    C. Hemangioma
    D. Myxoma
51. Commonest benign bone tumour is :
    A. Bone cyst
    B. Chondroma
    C. Chordoma
    D. Osteoid osteoma
52. In a 8 year old child the least common cause of lytic bone lesion in proximal femur :
    A. Plasmacytoma
    B. Histiocytoma
    C. Metastasis
    D. Brown tumour

Ans.	42. A	43. B	44. A	45. B	46. A	47. D
	48. A	49. B	50. B	51. D	52. A	

53.   Osteosarcoma differs from myositis ossificans by radiology :
       A. Location
       B. Infection is caused
       C. Shape of swelling
       D. Peripheral field of differentiation

54.   Osseous metastasis is most common if tumour is in :
       A. Bronchus   B. Colon
       C. Pancreas   D. Adrenal

55.   Treatment of choice of a solitary bony cyst is :
       A. Antibiotics
       B. Amputation
       C. Curettage+filling with bone chips
       D. Radiotherapy

56.   Most common lesion of hand is :
       A. Enchondroma   B. Synovioma
       C. Exostosis   D. Osteoclastoma

57.   Simple bone cyst contains :
       A. Blood   B. Clear fluid
       C. Thick gelatinous fluid   D. Cartilage lobules

58.   The symptom of pain from an ostseoid osteoma that first brings the
       patient to see a physician usually has history of duration of :
       A. One month   B. One month to one year
       C. Six month to two years   D. Two to five years
       E. Over five years

59.   Solitary myeloma may only be diagnosed when :
       A. There is reverse A/G ratio
       B. Electrophoresis shows abnormal globulins
       C. Bone marrow studies show a high percent of plasma cells
       D. All tests are normal except the direct biopsy

60.   Commonest site of multiple myeloma :
       A. Skull   B. Ribs
       C. Vertebra   D. Long bones
       E. Pelvis

61.   "Onion skin" layering of periosteal new bone by x-ray in midshaft
       location of Ewing's sarcoma may be expected to be present in what
       percentage of cases ?
       A. 10%   B. 25%
       C. 50%   D. 75%
       E. Over 80%

Ans.	53. D	54. A	55. C	56. A	57. B	58. C
	59. D	60. D	61. E			

62.   Perpendicular bone spiculation may be expected to be present in the x-ray of a midshaft Ewing's sarcoma in what percentage of cases ?
   A. 10%   B. 25%
   C. 50%   D. 75%
   E. Over 75%

63.   When Bence-Jones protein is found in urine, the diagnosis of myelomatosis is a in what percentage of cases ?
   A. 10%   B. 25%
   C. 50%   D. 75%
   E. Almost all of the cases

64.   The reversal of the A/G ratio in multiple myeloma is due to :
   A. An absolute decrease in the albumin fraction
   B. An absolute increase in the globulin fraction
   C. A relative reduction in the albumin
   D. A relative increase in the globulin
   E. A relative decrease in both with albumin affect most

65.   Which of the following symptoms are seen in a case of Ewing's tumour ?
   A. Raised temperature
   B. Palpable mass with pain locally
   C. Anaemia
   D. Leucocytosis
   E. All the above

66.   The cell of origin of Ewing's tumour, by recent proposition is :
   A. Endothelial
   B. Osteoblast
   C. Neuroectodermal
   D. Undifferentiated mesenchyme

67.   Common primary malignant tumour of bone is :
   A. Osteogenic sarcoma   B. Fibrosarcoma
   C. Liposarcoma   D. Chondrosarcoma
   E. None of the above

68.   All the following may mimic bone tumour, but which one is really a bone tumour ?
   A. Bone cyst   B. Fibrous dysplasia
   C. Hyperparathyrodism   D. Enchondroma

69.   Adamantinoma of limb bones are most frequently found in the :
   A. Humerus   B. Femur
   C. Tibia   D. Radius
   E. Ulna

Ans.	62. C	63. E	64. B	65. E	66. A	67. A
	68. D	69. C				

70. Which of these statements are incorrect concerning chondro-sarcoma ?
    A. It occurs mainly in middle-aged persons
    B. It is rare in children
    C. It has predilection for flat bones
    D. It does not metastasise to the lung

71. The most reliable method of obtaining a biopsy of a bone tumour is by means of :
    A. A trucut needle   B. A dril
    C. Open operation   D. A menghini needle

72. Treatment of painful bone metastasis is :
    A. Anticancer drugs   B. Hormones
    C. Radiotherapy   D. Immunotherapy

73. The commonest malignant bone tumour is :
    A. Myeloma   B. Osteosarcoma
    C. Ewing's sarcoma   D. Giant cell tumour

74. Which of the following bone tumours presents with pain first and swelling later on ?
    A. Osteoma   B. Chondroma
    C. Osteoclastoma   D. Osteosarcoma
    E. Ewing's tumour

75. Codman's tumour is :
    A. Osteosarcoma   B. Chondroblastoma
    C. Enchondroma   D. Fibrosarcoma

76. The treatment of choice in osteoclastoma in lower end of radius is :
    A. Radiotherapy
    B. Chemotherapy
    C. Amputation
    D. Cutting and filing with bone chips

77. Which has origin from diaphysis :
    A. Ewings sarcoma   B. Osteosarcoma
    C. Osteoclastoma   D. Chondroblastoma

78. The commonest malignant tumour in the rib is :
    A. Osteosarcoma   B. Fibrosarcoma
    C. Chondrosarcoma   D. Reticulum cell sarcoma

79. The radiological picture of fibrosarcoma may mimic :
    A. Osteolytic osteosarcoma
    B. Osteoclastoma
    C. An inflammatory lesion
    D. Any of the above

Ans.	70. D	71. C	72. C	73. A	74. D	75. B
	76. C	77. A	78. C	79. D		

W80. All are true regarding Ewing's tumor of bone except :
A. Arises from endothelial cells in bone marrow
B. Onion peel appearance on X-ray
C. Radiotherapy is treatment of choice
D. Forms differential diagnosis for osteomyelitis

81.   Treatment for haemangioma in bone is :
A. Excision
B. Currettage with bone grafting
C. Amputation
D. Masterly inactivity

82.   Treatment of fibrosarcoma is :
A. Surgery (wide excision) B. Surgery + Radiotherapy
C. Chemotherapy   D. Surgery+Chemotherapy

83.   The most radiosensitive tumor is :
A. Ewing's sarcoma   B. Fibrosarcoma
C. Osteosarcoma   D. Chondrosarcoma

84.   The tumour which bleed maximally is :
A. Fibrosarcoma   B. Leomyosarcoma
C. Osteosarcoma   D. Osteochondroma

85.   Osteoclastoma is common in age groups :
A. Below 10 years   B. 10-20 years
C. 20-40 years   D. All age group

86.   Osteoclastoma shows :
A. Expansile osteoblastic area in the diaphysis
B. Expansile osteolytic area in the diaphysis
C. Osteosclerotic area in the metaphysis
D. Osteolytic area in the metaphysis

87.   An eight-year old boy presents with progressive swelling around the knee joint of two months' duration following mild trauma. Local examination reveals an irregular bony swelling over the upper end of tibia, with raised local temperature and of variable consistency and illdefined margins. The most likely diagnosis :
A. Giant cell tumour   B. Ewing's sarcoma
C. Osteogenic sarcoma   D. Secondary metastasis

88.   Commonest carcinoma in 2nd to 3rd decade is :
A. Osteogenic sarcoma secondary to Paget's disease
B. Chondrosarcoma
C. Chondroblastoma
D. Primary osteogenic sarcoma

Ans.	80. NONE	81. A	82. A	83. A	84. B	85. C
	86. B	87. B	88. D			

89. Most common presentation of osteosarcoma is :
A. Soap bubble lesion
B. Localized pain & swelling
C. Formation of osteoid which does not calcify
D. Secondaries

90. Osteogenic sarcoma has all except :
A. New bone formation
B. Bone destruction
C. Periosteal elevation
D. Paget's disease predisposition
E. None of the above

91. For secondaries, uncommon site is :
A. Skull   B. Pelvis
C. Vertebrae   D. Femur

92. In carcinoma prostate with metastasis, which is raised :
A. ESR   B. Alkaline phosphatase
C. Acid phosphatase   D. Bilirubin

93. Enchondroma commonly arises from :
A. Ribs   B. Vertebra
C. Tibia   D. Phalanges

94. Carcinoma maxilla, stage T3N1. Treatment is :
A. Surgery+Radiation
B. Radiotherapy
C. Chemotherapy + radiotherapy
D. Only Chemotherapy

95. The treatment of enchondroma is :
A. Amputation
B. Irradiation
C. Local excision
D. Curettage and bone chip filling

96. Fish head appearance of the vertebral bodies is seen in all except :
A. Paget's disease   B. Rickets
C. Hypervitaminosis 'D' D. Osteoporosis

97. Pain in Osteoid osteoma is specifically relieved by :
A. Salicyiates   B. Narcotic analgesics
C. Radiation   D. Splinting

Ans.	89. B	90. E	91. D	92. C	93. D	94. A
	95. D	96. C	97. A			

Match the following :

98. **Morent Baker cyst :**
        a. Cyst with epithelised walls, hair and skin appendages

99. **Aneurysmal bone cyst :**
        b. Cyst due to retention of secretions of sebaceous glands

100. **Dermoid cyst :**
        c. Collection of synovial fluid in a sac between muscles or other tissues through a rent in capsule of the joint

101. **Sebaceous cyst :**
        d. Osteolytic lesion in a longbone or vertebral con sisting of blood filled spaces

102. **For secondaries, uncommon site is :**
  A. Skull   B. Pelvis
  C. Vertebrae   D. Femur

103. **Plaster of paris is :**
  A. Anhydrous calcium sulphate
  B. Used for immobilation
  C. First used in France
  D. All of above are true

104. **Most common primary tumour involving vertebra is :**
  A. Fibrosarcoma   B. Hodgkins disease
  C. Giant cell tumour   D. Multiple myeloma

105. **A child had a trivial fall and sustained a fracture to it's humerus. X-ray examination revealed lytic lesion. It could be :**
  A. Osteosarcoma   B. Osteoclastoma
  C. Osteomyeliti   D. Unicameral bone cyst

106. **The characteristic microscopic appearance of osteosarcoma is :**
  A. Osteoid formation
  B. Osteoblast formation with pleomorphism
  C. Osteoclast predominance
  D. Osteolytic lesions

107. **A women with fracture pelvis with pelvic hematoma, not passed urine since trauma ——C/I is :**
  A. Pass indwelling urethral catheter
  B. P.R. Examination
  C. IV fluids
  D. IV pyelography

Ans.	98. C	99. D	100. A	01. B	102. D	103. D
	104. D	105. D	106. A	107. A		

108. **Metastasis to bone is most common with following thyroid tumor :**
    - A. Follicular
    - B. Papillary
    - C. Medullary
    - D. Hurthle cell

109. **Age wise true for bone tumours :**
    - A. Osteosarcoma 6th decade
    - B. Multiple myeloma 5th decade
    - C. Chondrosarcoma 1st decade
    - D. Giant cell tumour 60-70 years

110. **Commonest tumour of jaw is :**
    - A. Ameloblastoma
    - B. Osteoma
    - C. Squamous cell carcinoma
    - D. Osteosarcoma

111. **Rare site of metastasis in Bone :**
    - A. Skull
    - B. Spine
    - C. Upper end of Humerus
    - D. Below elbow & Knees

112. **Ivory vertebrae are seen in :**
    - A. Osteosarcoma
    - B. Osteoclastoma
    - C. Chondrosarcoma
    - D. Hemangioma

113. **Most common benign tumor of temperomandibular joint is :**
    - A. Osteoma
    - B. Osteochondroma
    - C. Unicameral bone cyst
    - D. Granuloma

114. **Chordoma is seen in all except :**
    - A. Clivus
    - B. Sacrum
    - C. Vertebral bodies
    - D. Ribs

115. **True about Ewing's sarcoma is all except :**
    - A. 5% cases reveals t (11-22)
    - B. Arise from medullary cavity of tubular bone
    - C. Arise from diaphysis
    - D. N-myc chromosome

116. **Radiological features of Ewing sarcoma least mimics following except :**
    - A. Osteomyelitis
    - B. Rheumatoid arthritis
    - C. Recticulum cell carcinoma
    - D. Osteogenic sarcoma

117. **Osteotrophic secondaries are all except :**
    - A. Ca prostate
    - B. Ca lung
    - C. Ca breast
    - D. Multiple myeloma

Ans.	108. D	109. B	110. A	111. D	112. D	113. B
	114. D	115. B	16. A	117. A		

118. **Tumour most commonly metastatizing to bone :**
    A. Fibrosarcoma
    B. Synovioma
    C. Angiosarcoma
    D. Myoma

119. **In skull X-ray, lytic bevelled lesions are seen, most likely cause is :**
    A. Multiple myeloma
    B. Eosinophilic granuloma
    C. Osteosarcoma
    D. Metastasis

120. **Secondary tumour in osteochondroma is :**
    A. Osteosarcoma
    B. Chondrosarcoma
    C. Osteochondrosarcoma
    D. Malignant histiocytoma

121. **Babu, 19 yrs has small circumscribed sclerotic swelling over diaphysis of femur bone; Diagnosis is :**
    A. Osteoclastoma
    B. Osteosarcoma
    C. Ewings sarcoma
    D. Osteoid osteoma

122. **Babloo, age 10 yeas, presents with fracture of humerus. X-ray reveals lesion at the upper end. Likely condition is :**
    A. Unicameral bone cyst
    B. Osteosarcoma
    C. Giant cell tumour
    D. Osteochondroma

123. **Radiotherapy is the treatment of choice in :**
    A. Ewing's sarcoma
    B. Osteosarcoma
    C. Osteoclastoma
    D. Synovial sarcoma

124. **Onion skinning in Ewing's sarcoma represents :**
    A. Periodicity in growth of tumor
    B. Attempts of periosteum to limit tumor growth
    C. Haemorrhages inside the rapidly growing tumor
    D. Compression of tumor over soft tissues

125. **A 19-year-old patient came with pain the his right femur. The X-ray showed a lytic lesion surrounded by a sclerotic zone in the diaphysis. The diagnosis is most probably :**
    A. Ewing's sarcoma
    B. Osteoid osteoma
    C. Osteoclastoma
    D. Osteoblastoma

126. **Inversion injury of the foot is associated with damage to all the following except :**
    A. Lateral malleolus
    B. Base of 5th metatarsal bone
    C. Sustentaculum tali tear
    D. Extensor digitorum brevis

127. **Patellar tendon bearing POP cast is to be applied in :**
    A. Femoral fracture
    B. Patellar fracture
    C. Tibial fracture
    D. Medial malleolar fracture

Ans.	118. A	119. B	120. B	121. D	122. A	123. A
	124. B	125. B	126. D	127. C		

128. A 11-year old boy presented with the complaints of pain in the right arm near the shoulder. X-ray examination revealed an expansile lytic lesion in the upper third of humerus. The most likely diagnosis is :
    A. Giant cell tumour
    B. Unicameral bone cyst
    C. Osteochondroma
    D. Parosteal osteosarcoma

129. Management plan for osteogenic sarcoma of the lower end of femur must include?
    A. Radiotherapy-amputation-chemotherapy
    B. Surgery alone
    C. Chemotherapy-limb salvage surgery-chemotherapy
    D. Chemotherapy + radiotherapy

130. Widespread patchy sclerosis of the skeleton can be seen in except :
    A. Mast cell reticulosis   B. Carcinoma of the breast
    C. Neuroblastoma   D. Fluorosis
    E. Myeloid metaplasia

131. Onion peel appearance is seen in :
    A. Osteoclastoma   B. Chondrosarcoma
    C. Osteosarcoma   D. Ewings sarcoma

132. Lytic lesion in upper end of tibia is expansile and has soap - buble appearance :
    A. Osteoclastoma   B. Osteogenic Sarcoma
    C. Ewing's Sarcoma   D. Osteoblastoma

133. Earliest bone metastasis can be detected by :
    A. Compound tomography
    B. Plain X - rays
    C. Radio - isoscope bone scan
    D. Tomography

134. Which of the following does not describe chondro-blastoma :
    A. Non calcifying
    B. Eccentric
    C. Epiphyseal location
    D. Simulates giant cell tumour of bone

135. Commonest cause of punched out lesions in phalanges is :
    A. Enchondroma   B. Chondrosarcoma
    C. Aneurysmal bone cyst D. Multiple myeloma

136. Sun-ray appeerence is seen in following except :
    A. Multiple myeloma   B. Sturge-Weber syndrome
    C. Osteogenic sarcomas D. Meningioma

Ans.	128. B	129. C	130. C	131. D	132. A	133. C
	134. A	135. A	136. B			

137. **Mutton-leg like gross appearance is seen in :**
   A. Osteosarcoma   B. Osteoclastoma
   C. Chondrosarcoma   D. Ewing's sarcoma

138. **Osteoclastic secondaries are seen in following :**
   A. Rectum   B. Liver
   C. Breasts   D. Prostate

139. **Which of the following tumour originates from diaphysis :**
   A. Ewing's sarcoma   B. Osteosarcoma
   C. Osteoclastoma   D. Chondrosarcoma

140. **Codman's tumour is :**
   A. Osteosarcoma   B. Chondroblastoma
   C. Enchondroma   D. Fibrosarcoma

141. **Osteosarcomas spread by :**
   A. Permeation in lymphatics
   B. Embolisation in lymphatics
   C. Embolism in vessels
   D. Permeation in vessels

142. **In the female, Bone metastases most often orginate from carcinoma of the :**
   A. Breast   B. Endometrium
   C. Ovary   D. Cervix

143. **The commonest sarcoma of man (excluding lymphomas) :**
   A. Liposarcoma   B. Fibrosarcoma
   C. Osteosarcoma   D. Angiosarcoma

144. **True about osteosarcoma are all except :**
   A. Seen commonly in young males
   B. Predisposed in Paget's disease
   C. Predisposed in fibrous dysplasia
   D. 5 year survival is 50%

145. **Blood borne metastasis is unusual of :**
   A. Osteosarcoma   B. Medullary carcinoma brast
   C. Chriocarcinoma   D. Renal cell carcinoma

146. **Bone tumour which is hormone dependent :**
   A. Osteogenic sarcoma   B. Ewings sarcoma
   C. Osteoclastoma   D. Fibrous dysplasia

147. **Radiation is least likely to cause :**
   A. Fibrosarcoma
   B. Fibrosarcoma + Oesteosarcoma
   C. Chondrosarcoma
   D. Chondroblastoma

Ans.	137. A	138. D	139. A	140. B	141. C	142. A
	143. C	144. C	145. B	146. D	147. A	

148. **The commonest malignant bone tumour is :**
    A. Multiple myeloma   B. Osteosarcoma
    C. Ewing's sarcoma   D. Giant cell tumour

149. **Which of the following is a true bone tumour :**
    A. Aneurysmal bone cyst B. Fibrous dysplasia
    C. Enchordroma   D. All of the above

150. **Bone tumor arising from Epiphysis is :**
    A. Osteogenic sarcoma   B. Chondromyxoid fibroma
    C. Ewing's sarcoma   D. Giant cell tumor

151. **Giant cells are seen in all of the following bone tumors except :**
    A. Osteoclastoma   B. Benign chondroclastoma
    C. Chondromyxoid fibromaD. Osteoid ostroma

152. **Presence of Osteoid without mineralization is seen in :**
    A. Rickets   B. Scurvy
    C. Osteopetrosis   D. Paget's disease

153. **Histology of Ewing's sarcoma shows small round   cells. These cells are filled with which of the   following :**
    A. Iron   B. Fat
    C. Mucin   D. Glycogen

154. **A 50 year old patient presents with a lesion in the midline involving the sacrum which is sclerotic. What is the likely diagnosis :**
    A. Osteosarcoma   B. Chordoma
    C. Metastasis   D. Chondrosarcoma

155. **Bone tumor most commonly arising from pelvis :**
    A. Chondiosarcoma   B. Osteogenic sarcoma
    C. Ewing's sarcoma   D. Giant cell tumor

156. **The tumor most commonly metastasizing to bone is :**
    A. Neuroblastoma   B. Wilm's tumor
    C. Glioma   D. Sarcoma

157. **A 12 year old girl complains of pain persisting in his left leg. For several weeks with a low grade fever. A radiograph   reveals a mass in the diaphyseal region of the left femur with overlying cortical erosion and soft tissue extension. A biopsy of the lesion shows numerous small round cells, rich in PAS positive diastase sensitive granules. The most likely histological diagnosis is :**
    A. Osteogenic sarcoma.
    B. Osteoblastoma.
    C. Ewing's sarcoma.
    D. Chondroblastoma.

158. **All are giant cell lesions of bone except :**
    A. Aneurysmal bone cyst B. Chandroblastoma
    C. Brown tumor   D. Chondroma

Ans.	148. A	149. C	150. D	151. D	152. A	153. D
	154. B	155. A	156. A	157. C	158. D	

MAXILLO FACIAL SYSTEM

1. **The most common malignant lesion of parotid gland is :**
    A. Mucoepidermoid carcinoma
    B. Adenocystic carcinoma
    C. Acinar cell adenocarcinoma
    D. Anaplastic adenocarcinoma
    E. Squamous cell carcinoma
2. **Parotid tumour which spreads perineurally is :**
    A. Mucoepidermoid carcinoma
    B. Epidermoid carcinoma
    C. Carcinoma in pleomorphic adenoma
    D. Adenoid cystic carcinoma
3. **Regarding aphthous stomatitis which of the following is incorrect ?**
    A. It is confined to infant
    B. It can be due to a virus
    C. It can caused by Monilia
    D. It can be caused by Candida
4. **Leukoplakia of the tongue is not associated with :**
    A. A jagged tooth   B. Smoking
    C. Dyskeratosis   D. Aspergillus niger
5. **Hot spot on Tc Scan in parotid in :**
    A. Adenolymphoma   B. Mixed parotid tumour
    C. Calculus   D. Mumps
    E. Sjorgren's disease
6. **Most common salivary gland tumor in a child is :**
    A. Mucoepidermoid
    B. Adenolymphone
    C. Acinic cell
    D. A denoid cystic carcinoma
7. **Most common tumour of minor salivary glands is :**
    A. Epidermoid carcinoma
    B. Mixed tumour
    C. Squamous cell carcinoma
    D. Epilethioma
8. **Commonest parotid tumour is:**
    A. Pleomorphic adenoma B. Warthin's tumour
    C. Adenoid cystic ca   D. Secondaries

Ans.	1. A	2. D	3. A	4. D	5. A	6. A
	7. A	8. A				

9. **Regarding CA lip not true is:**
   A. Lower lip commonly involved
   B. Early cases surgery and radiotherapy curative
   C. Early metastasis to lymph nodes
   D. Kiss cancer type

10. **Commonest site for carcinoma tongue is :**
    A. Lateral margin of ant. 2/3
    B. Tip of the tongue
    C. Dorsum posteriroly
    D. Ventral

11. **A patient with cheek cancer has a tumour of 2.5 cm located close to and involving the lowwer alveolus. A single mobile homolateral lymphnode measured 6 cm is palpable. The TNM stage is :**
    A. T1,N1M0   B. T2,N2,M0
    C. T2,N1,M0   D. T4,N2,M0

12. **In the treatment of cancer cheek using a single drug, the best results are obtained with :**
    A. Cisplatinum   B. Methotrexate
    C. Bleomycin   D. Endoxon

13. **Mixed parotid tumour arises from :**
    A. Epithelium
    B. Epithelium + Mesenchyme
    C. Mesenchyme
    D. None of the above

14. **Regarding carcinoma of tongue which is incorrect :**
    A. Starts as painless ulcer
    B. May present as a fissure
    C. Common site is posterior one third of tongue
    D. In late cases, pain may radiate

15. **Tumours of the palate include the following except :**
    A. Ectopic salivary tumour
    B. A carcinoma of the maxillary antrum
    C. An alveolar abscess of the incisors
    D. A transitional-cell carcinoma

16. **Ca buccal mucosa metastasized to :**
    A. Submandibular nodes
    B. Jugulodiagastric nodes
    C. Jugulo omohyoid nodes
    D. Brain

Ans.	9. C	10. A	11. C	12. A	13. B	14. C
	15. D	16. B				

17. **A Warthin's tumour is :**
    A. An adenolymphoma of the parotid gland
    B. A pleomorphic adenoma of the parotid
    C. A cylindroma
    D. A carcinoma of the parotid

18. **Which carcinoma does not belong to oral cancer :**
    A. Posterior 1/3 of tongue   B. Hard palate
    C. Cheek   D. Tongue anterior 1/3

19. **Warthin's tumor is best treated by :**
    A. Superficial parotidectomy
    B. Enucleation
    C. Radiotherapy
    D. Chemotherapy

20. **In carcinoma of tip of tongue, lymph nodes not involved are :**
    A. Juglodiagastric   B. Retropharyngeal
    C. Submandibular   D. None of the above

21. **Epidermoid carcinoma of following has best prog- nosis :**
    A. Lip   B. Buccal muosa
    C. Palate   D. Tongue

22. **Warthin's tumour is :**
    A. Malignant
    B. Rapiadly
    C. Gives a hot pertechnetate scan
    D. Cold pertenchnetate scan

23. **Cancer tongue may have all the following features   except :**
    A. Pain in the ear   B. Pain in swallowing
    C. Ankyloglossis   D. Nasal regurgitation

24. **A 60-year old female presents with a non-healing ulcer with raised edges on the face four years duration, without any significant lymph node enlargement. The most likely diagnosis is :**
    A. Basal cell carcinoma   B. Epidermoid carcinoma
    C. Malignant melanoma   D. Mycosis fungoides

25. **2.5 cm involvement of oral cavity carcinoma with contralateral mobile lymph node, staging is :**
    A. T2N2   B. T2N3
    C. T1N1   D. T2

26. **In radical neck dissection, which nerve is sometimes sacrificed :**
    A. 9   B. 10
    C. 11   D. 12

Ans.	17. A	18. B	19. A	20. B	21. A	22. C
	23. D	24. A	25. A	26. C		

27. **Carcinoma of lip is histologically :**
   A. Squamous cell ca B. Adenoca
   C. Basal cell ca D. None

28. **The most common tumor in the mandible is :AIIMS 2001**
   A. Osteoblastoma B. Ameloblastoma
   C. Squamous cell carcinoma D. Lymphoma

29. **A 55yr old man presents with 1x2 cm ulcer in the right lateral border of tongue. Biopsy from the lesion revealed well-differentiated squamous cell carcinoma. The most appropriate management is :**
   A. Interstitial brachytherapy
   B. External beam irradiation + immunotherapy
   C. Laser ablation
   D. Chemotherapy

30. **An edentulous patient has carcinoma of the oral cavity infiltrating into the alveolar margin. Which of the following would not be indicated in managing the case :**
   A. Segmental mandibulectomy
   B. Marginal mandibulectomy with removal of the outer table
   C. Marginal mandibulectomy with removal of upper half mandible
   D. Radiotherapy

31. **Which one of the following odontomas is locally invasive malignant tuor :**
   A. Odontogenic myxoma
   B. Fibromatous epulis
   C. Dentigerous cyst
   D. Ameloblastoma

| Ans. | 27. A | 28. C | 29. A | 30. B | 31. D |

NECK & BREAST

NECK

1. **Most common type of parathyroid adenoma is :**
    A. Clear cell adenoma   B. Chief cell adenoma
    C. Oxyphil cell adenoma D. A + B
    E. B + C

2. **Medullary carcinoma of thyroid associated with each of the following except :**
    A. Prostaglandins
    B. Serotonin
    C. Calcitonin
    D. Multiple endocrine adenomatosis
    E. Better prognosis than papillary carcinoma

3. **Cystic hygroma is a kind of :**
    A. Lymphoma   B. Lymphangioma
    C. Hemangioma   D. Capillary angioma

4. **FNAC is not of much use in which thyroid pathology ? :**
    A. Papillary carcinoma   B. Follicular carcinoma
    C. Medullary carcinoma   D. Thyroiditis

5. **Thyroid carcinoma with best prognosis is :**
    A. Papillary carcinoma   B. Follicular carcinoma
    C. Anaplastic type   D. Medullary type

6. **All of the following are used in effectively treating recurrent thyroid cancer except :**
    A. Chemotherapy   B. Further surgery
    C. High doses of I131 D. High doses of thyroxine

7. **Hypocalcemia in immediate post operative period following excision of parathyroid adenoma is due to :**
    A. Increased calcitonin   B. Stress
    C. Hypercalciuria   D. Increased uptake by bone

8. **Multiple cold nodules in a thyroid scan is a feature of :**
    A. Multi nodular goitre
    B. Multicentric papillary Ca.
    C. Grave's disease
    D. Hashimoto's thyoiditis

Ans.	1. B	2. E	3. B	4. B	5. A	6. A
	7. D	8. A				

9. **Secondaries in the neck with no obvious primary malignancy is most often due to :**
   A. Ca. Larynx   B. Ca. Nasopharyx
   C. Ca. Thyroid   D. Ca. Stomach

10. **Treatment of choice for cold nodule in thyroid is :**
    A. I^{131}
    B. Hemithyroidectomy
    C. Subtotal thyroidectomy
    D. Wait and watch

11. **The type of Thyroid Ca. which produces high level of serum calcitonin   is :**
    A. Follicular   B. Papillary
    C. Anaplastic   D. Medullary

12. **Medullary carcinoma of thyroid arises from :**
    A. Follicular cell lining
    B. Interfollicular C-cells
    C. Parathyroid cells in thyroid
    D. Parathyroid gland

13. **Calcitonin is a marker in serum for :**
    A. Anaplastic carcinoma B. Medullary carcinoma
    C. Papillary carcinoma   D. Follicular carcinoma

14. **I^{131} scan of thyroid is useful to :**
    A. Estimate function   B. Detect cold nodules
    C. Diagnose carcinoma   D. All the above

15. **Retrotracheal extension of thyroid mass can be recognised by :**
    A. X-ray neck   B. C.T.scan
    C. Barium swallow   D. Ultrasound

16. **Occult carcinoma of the thyroid is seen in :**
    A. Papillary carcinoma B. Medullary
    C. Anaplastic   D. Hurthle-cell carcinoma

17. **A cold nodule of the thyroid may be due to the following except :**
    A. Cyst of the thyroid
    B. Degeneration in a nodule
    C. Carcinoma
    D. Parenchymatous goitre

18. **Which of the following is inappropriate to cystic hygroma ?**
    A. It is a type of cavernous haemangioma
    B. It can be the earliest swelling of the neck to appear in life
    C. It can obstruct labour
    D. It is brilliantly translucent

Ans.	9. B	10. B	11. D	12. B	13. B	14. B
	15. B	16. A	17. D	18. A		

19. **The 'Potato's tumour of the neck is a :**
    A. Sternomastoid tumour   B. Carotid body tumour
    C. Thyroid tumour   D. Parotid tumour

20. **In non-endemic zones, solitary nodule of the thyroid is result of:**
    A. Thyroditis   B. Adenoma
    C. Follicular carcinoma   D. Colloid goitre

21. **Following are true about thyroid tumor except :**
    A. Malignant tumors are solid in USS
    B. 40-50% malignat nodules are cold in isotops scanning
    C. FNAC biopsy is not diagnostic
    D. Calcitonin is a tumor marker for medullary Ca thyroid

22. **Which of the following is not an histological type of carcinoma of the thyroid?**
    A. Transitional   B. Papillary
    C. Anaplastic   D. Medullary

23. **Sternomastoid tumour appears :**
    A. Congenitally   B. Soon after birth
    C. In first week of life   D. At the age of 2—6 weeks

24. **Regarding carotid body tumour, which of the following is not true :**
    A. In increases gradually
    B. It responds very well to radiotherapy
    C. It is usually unilateral
    D. Vertical movements are not possible whereas it can be moved horizontally
    E. None of the above

25. **With which of the following medullary carcinoma of thyroid is associated :**
    A. Cushing's syndrome   B. Carcinoid syndrome
    C. Phaeochromocytoma   D. Hyperparathyroidism
    E. All of the above

26. **Treatment of cystic hygroma is :**
    A. Surgical excision   B. Injection of sclerosants
    C. Irradiation   D. Majesty inactivity

27. **Best treatment of anaplastic carcinoma of thyroid is :**
    A. Chemotherapy   B. Subtotal thyroidectomy
    C. Total thyroidectomy   D. External radiation

28. **The special danger of a carotid body tumour is that :**
    A. It recurs after excision
    B. It is blended with the carotid artery

Ans.	19. D	20. C	21. A	22. B	23. B	24. B
	25. E	26. A	27. D			

C. It is blended with the external jungular vein

D. It is radioresistant

29. **A solitary nodule in thyroid in a middle aged lady is :**

A. Carcinoma   B. Multinodular goitre

C. Adenoma   D. Physiological goitre

30. **A multiloculated translucent swelling in posterior triangle of neck of a child :**

A. Cystic hygroma   B. Thyroglossal cyst

C. Hemangiomas   D. Branchial cyst

31. **Metastatic calcium deposits are seen in :**

A. Thyroid neoplasm   B. Parathyroid neoplasm

C. Thyrotoxicosis   D. Thymoma

32. **Example of radiation induced Ca is :**

A. Papillary carcinoma thyroid

B. Follicular carcinma thyroid

C. Lymphoma

D. Hepatoma

E. Seminoma

33. **Treatment of choice in well-differentiated thyroid carcinoma :**

A. Radio iodine

B. Near total thyroidectomy

C. Subtotal thyroidectomy

D. Radiation

E. Total thyroparathyroidectomy

34. **Among following most common cause of solitary thyroid nodule is :**

A. Adenomatous goitre   B. Follicular adenoma

C. Papillary adenoma   D. Papillary carcinoma

35. **All of the following regarding papillary carcinoma thyroid is true except :**

A. Multicentric origin

B. Secondaries to lymph nodes

C. Slowly growing

D. Bony metastasis in early stage

36. **'Brown Tumors' are seen in :**

A. Secondaries of bones   B. Hyperparathyroidism

C. Hypothyroidism   D. Adrenal tumors

Ans.	28. B	29. C	30. A	31. B	32. A	33. B
	34. B	35. D	36. B			

37. Of the following methods which one is the most sensitive for detecting parathyroid adenomas ?
   A. Barium cine esophagography
   B. Selenomethionine scanning
   C. Thallium-Technitium Substraction Scanning
   D. Inferior thyroid arteriography

38. Papillary Carcinoma of thyroid is associated with following except:
   A. Psammoma Bodies
   B. Papillary processes
   C. Follicular pattern with papillary processes
   D. Amyloid stroma

39. Medullary carcinoma of thyroid is characterized by following except :
   A. Secretes calcitonin   B. Hereditary in nature
   C. Amyloid stroma is seen   D. Hormone dependent

40. Thyroid carcinoma with pulsating vescular skeletal metastasis is :
   A. Papillary   B. Anaplastic
   C. Follicular   D. Medullary

41. Which is the least common in thyroid scan in case of follicular carcinoma :
   A. Hot   B. Warm
   C. Cold   D. Isothermic

42. Medullary carcinoma thyroid is associated with :
   A. Pheochromocytoma   B. Pituitary carcinoma
   C. Carcinoid syndrome D. Testicular tumour
   E. Neuroblastoma

43. Which is not true regarding carotid body tumour :
   A. Is radio resistant
   B. Is a non-chromafin paraganglioma
   C. May have massive bleeding
   D. Surgical removal is treatment of choice

44. The following are true regarding solitary nodule of Thyroid except one :
   A. 20% are malignant
   B. More than 50% of cold nodules are malignant
   C. FNAC has become established as the investigation of choice
   D. More common in women
   E. The only indication for isotope scanning is combination of toxicity and nodularity

Ans.	37. C	38. D	39. D	40. C	41. D	42. A
	43. D	44. B				

45. **Kalloo, 45 years, presents with a swelling in the thyroid gland and a lymphnode in the neck. Aspiration of the node shows amyloid material. What is the management of choice for this patient :**
   A. Hemithyroidectomy with neck dissection
   B. Total thyroidectomy, with neck dissection
   C. Total thyroidectomy with neck irradiation
   D. Hemithyroidectomy

46. **Risk factors for thyroid carcinoma are following except :**
   A. Family H/o papillary Ca   B. Family H/o medullary Ca
   C. Low dose irridiation   D. None of the above

47. **Ocult thyroid malignancies are usually :**
   A. Follicular   B. Medullary
   C. Papillary   D. Anaplastic

48. **Which one of the following statements regarding medullary carcinoma of thyroid is correct ?**
   A. Total thyroidectomy is curative.
   B. It is TSH dependent.
   C. Radioactive iodine is useful in the treatment.
   D. Chemotherapy and total thyroidectomy are curative.

49. **Which malignancy would occur in prolonged multinodular goiter ?**
   A. Papillary carcinoma   B. Follicular carcinoma
   C. Anaplastic carcinoma   D. Medullary carcinoma

50. **A patient with carcinoma of the tongue was found to have lymph nodes in the lower neck. The treatment of choice for the lymph nodes is :**
   A. Radical neck dissection B. Chemotherapay
   C. Tele radiotherapy   D. Local excision

51. **Parathyroid adenoma most commonly involves :**
   A. Inferior glands
   B. Superior glands
   C. Substance of thyroid
   D. Arises from ectopic parathyroid in mediastinum

BREAST

52. **In breast cancer, stage T.N.M. indicats :**
   A. Tumour more than 2 cm diameter with axillary nodes
   B. Tumour <2 cm, no nodes, no metastases
   C. Tumour fixed to chest wall, no axillary nodes, no metastases
   D. Fixed to pectoralis, no axillary nodes

53. **Prognosis in cancer of the breast is most favourable in :**
   A. Upper outer quadrant B. Lower outer quadrant
   C. Upper inner quadrant D. Lower inner quadrant

Ans.	45. B	46. A	47. C	48. A	49. B	50. A
	51. A	52. B	53. A			

54. **In Paget's disease nipple, secretions is mainly :**
    A. Mucous material   B. Water
    C. Blood   D. All of the above

55. **Paget's disease of nipple is treated by :**
    A. Radiotherapy
    B. Biopsy and simple mastectomy
    C. Radical mastectomy
    D. Chemotherapy

56. **Most common regime used in Ca breast :**
    A. CMF   B. CAV
    C. CHOP   D. PEB

57. **Detection of lipoma like swelling in breast is indicative of :**
    A. Presence of true lipoma   B.   Fibroadenosis
    C. Underlying cancer   D. A benign condition
    E. None of the above

58. **Lymphnode which is first to be involved in carcinoma breast :**
    A. Pectoral group   B. Internal mammary
    C. Apical   D. Central
    E. Supra clavicular

59. **Massive swellings of the breast include the following except :**
    A. Cystosarcoma phylloides
    B. Atrophic scirrhous carcinoma
    C. Diffuse hypertrophy
    D. Giant fibroadenoma

60. **The following are clinical signs supporting an early diagnosis of carcinoma of the breast :**
    A. A prickling sensation in a breast lump
    B. Peau d' Orange
    C. Brawny arm
    D. Cancer en Cruisse

61. **Regarding follow-up of patients with carcinoma of the breast except :**
    A. It is unnecessary for a surgeon to follow up his patients with carcinoma of the breast after operation. It is done by other specialities
    B. A rectal examination may be necessary
    C. The liver should be examined
    D. X-ray of the chest is a routine follow up examiantion

62. **In TNM classification, stage II carcinoma breast is :**
    A. T2N2M0   B. T2N1M0
    C. T3N1M0   D. T1N0M0

Ans.	54. B	55. B	56. A	57. D	58. A	59. B
	60. A	61. A	62. B			

63. **Carcinoma breast is common in :**
    A. Cystic disease   B. Duct ectasia
    C. Epithelial hyperplasia D. Sclerosing adenosis

64. **In radical mastectomy, the structure to be ligated is :**
    A. Axillary vein   B. Axillary artery
    C. Innominte vein   D. Phrenic nerve

65. **"Breast mouse" is found in cases of :**
    A. Bite by a mouse   B. Hard fibroadenoma
    C. Soft fibroadenoma   D. Papillary cystadenoma
    E. Fibroadenosis

66. **The early sign suggesive of carcinoma breast is :**
    A. Peaud's orange
    B. Brawny arm
    C. Breast lump with pricking sensation
    D. Hyperpyrexia

67. **Which of the following are indicative of inoperability in patients with breast cancer except :**
    A. Inflammatory cancer
    B. Satellite skin nodules
    C. Parasternal nodules
    D. Involved axillary lymphnodes

68. **Radical mastectomy is contraindicated in :**
    A. Peaud' orange
    B. Breast lesion with appearance of shotty axillary lymphnodes
    C. Blood stained nipple discharge
    D. Acute inflammatory reaction

69. **Which of the following is least frequent site for breast metastasis?**
    A. Lung   B. Liver
    C. Bone   D. Contralateral breast

70. **A 50-year old female presents with a fungating carcinoma of the breast, 8 cm in diameter. Mobile 1 cm diameter nodes are palpable in the ipsilateral axilla. Chest X-ray and bone scan are normal. The treatment of choice for her would be :**
    A. Simple mastectomy with axillary clearance and postoperative chemotherapy
    B. Simple mastectomy with axillary node sampling and postoperative radiotherapy; chemotherapy if nodes are positive
    C. Radiotherapy to breast and chemotherapy
    D. Radical mastectomy and chemotherapy

Ans.	63. C	64. B	65. B	66. C	67. D	68. D
	69. D	70. B				

71. Of the operations listed, the interests of a patient with a stage III carcinoma of the breast are best served by :
   A. A radical mastectomy
   B. A super-radical mastectomy
   C. Simple mastectomy
   D. Lumpectomy

72. A 50-year old woman was operated for left radical mastectomy. During physical examination she was asked to face a wall and push hard against it with both hands outstretched. It was noticed that inferior angle and medial border of the left Scapula projected medially. Which nerve was injured during the left mastectomy?
   A. Nerve to deltoid
   B. Nerve to serratus anterior
   C. Nerve to trapezius
   D. Nerve to lattismus dorsi

73. A 40-year old female presents with a 9-months hisotry of a swelling in the outer quadrant of the breast. It is 3 cm diameter and is not attached to the skin or deep fascia. Lymph nodes are enlarged and mobile in the axilla. There are no supraclavicular lymph nodes. Chest X-ray is normal. Biopsy showed scirrhous carcinoma. The correct course of treatment in this case would be :
   A. Simple mastectomy and radiotherapy
   B. Radical mastectomy
   C. Radical mastectomy and radiotherapy
   D. Radiotherapy

74. The diagnosis of breast carcinoma is established by local excision of the palpable lump, and resdual or multicentric cancer may be demonstrated in —— of mastectomy specimens.
   A. 10%   B. 20%
   C. 30%   D. 60%

75. A 40-year old lady underwent radical mastectomy for a 2 cm carcinma of the breast. Histopathology of axillary nodes removed did not show any secondaries. The most appropriate future line of management would be :
   A. Periodic follow up for any recurence and treatment thereof
   B. Radiotherapy
   C. Chemotherapy
   D. Hormone therapy

76. Secondary deposits from carcinoma breast are commonest in :
   A. Lung   B. Liver
   C. Brain   D. Bone

| Ans. | 71. B | 72. B | 73. A | 74. D | 75. A | 76. D |

77. **Risk factor for carcinoma breast is :**
   A. Fibroadenoma on the side
   B. Sister dead from cancer breast
   C. Jewish origin
   D. All of the above

78. **Greenish discharge from the nipple is suggestive of :**
   A. Carcinoma   B. Duct papilloma
   C. Duct carcinoma   D. Fibroadenosis

79. **Treatment of choice in duct papilloma is :**
   A. Radiotherapy   B. Microdochectomy
   C. Chemotherapy   D. No treatment

80. **Most common type of carcinoma breast is :**
   A. Paget's   B. Lobular
   C. Comedo   D. Ductal

81. **Paget's disease of the breast has all of the following except :**
   A. Nipple scaling
   B. Sanguinous nipple discharge
   C. Constitutes 10% of all breast carcinomas
   D. Arises from the ductal tissue above the nipple

82. **Adrenelectomy in carcinoma breast is indicated when the following is involved :**
   A. Liver   B. Lung
   C. Bone   D. Lymphnode

83. **In Axillary tail carcinoma, treatment is :**
   A. Simple mastectomy   B. Radical mastectomy
   C. Extended mastectomy D. Chemotherapy

84. **In carcinoma breast with axillary lymph node involvement and partial mastectomy done in the past, next treatment is :**
   A. Radiotherapy   B. Chemotherapy
   C. Oophrectomy   D. Hypophysectomy

85. **Commonest site of carcinoma breast is :**
   A. Upper and outer quadrant
   B. Upper and medial quadrant
   C. Lower and medial quadrant
   D. Lower and lateral quadrant

86. **Paget's disease of the breast is :**
   i.   A premalignant condition
   ii. A disease primarily involving the nipple
   iii. Treated by simple mastectomy

Ans.	77. B	78. D	79. B	80. D	81. C	82. C
	83. B	84. A	85. A	86. C		

Of these statements
A. (i) (ii) and (iii) are correct
B. (i) and (ii) are correct
C. (ii) and (iii) are correct
D. (i) and (iii) are correct

87. Chemotherapy in carcinoma breast is particularly useful in one of the following :
A. Local lesion (Primary)
B. Bony secondaries
C. Lymph node involvement
D. Visceral spread

88. One of these has a greater prognostic value in carcinoma breast :
A. Size of the tumour
B. Age of the patient
C. Presence of the pain
D. Involvement of lymph nodes

89. Blood stained discharge from the nipple is typical of :
A. Paget's disease of the nipple
B. Intra-ductal papilloma
C. Fibroadenosis   -
D. Filarial mastitits

90. The treatment of fibroadenoma of the breast is :
A. Simple mastectomy   B. Local excision
C. Observation   D. Radiotherapy

91. Which of the following rule out radical mastectomy for breast cancer :
A. Enlarged and fixed axillary nodes
B. Fixation of lesion to chest wall
C. Proven distant metastasis
D. Skin ulceration
E. All of the above

92. The least effective palliative treatment for advanced carcinoma of the male breast is :
A. Orchiectomy   B. Hormone therapy
C. Adrenalectomy   D. Hypophysectomy
E. Cytotoxic agents

93. Tumours of aberrant breast tissue are rare; in which of the following may an aberrant carcinoma present most frequently ?
A. Axilla   B. Infraclavicular region
C. Sternal area   D. Epigastrium
E. Close to xiphistrium

Ans.	87. D	88. D	89. B	90. B	91. E	92. B
	93. A					

94. **Prognosis in male breast Ca depends on :**
    A. Duration of disease   B. Ulceration of nipple
    C. Nipple discharge   D. L.N. Status

95. **Which of the following may not be considered "minimal" breast cancer ?**
    A. Duct cancer less 1 cm in outer quadrants
    B. Lobular carcinoma in situ
    C. Duct carcinoma less than 1 cm in inner quandrants
    D. Colloid carcinoma
    E. Early "paget's disease"

96. **Which of the following is true of cystosarcoma phylloides :**
    A. Small tumour   B. Locally invasive
    C. Highly malignant   D. Early metastasis

97. **Peau d' orange in carcinoma breast is due to :**
    A. Lymphatic blockage
    B. Invasion of ligament of Cooper
    C. Sweat gland blockage
    D. Lactiferous duct invasion

98. **Carcinoma breast which is most often bilateral is :**
    A. Medullary carcinoma
    B. Lobular carcinoma
    C. Ductal adenocarcinoma
    D. Paget's disease

99. **In the treatment of breast cancer, Tamoxifen is used in :**
    A. Pre-menopausal women
    B. Estrogen receptor positive tumor
    C. Presence of lymph nodes
    D. Presence of bone metastasis

100. **Treatment of choice in cystosarcoma phylloides is :**
    A. Simple mastectomy
    B. Modified Radical Mastectomy
    C. Radical mastectomy
    D. Lumpectomy

101. **Hypercalcemia in breast cancer is most often due to :**
    A. Tumor necrosis   B. Ectopic parathormone
    C. Bone Secondaries   D. Chest wall invasion

102. **Commonest cause of bleeding from nipple is :**
    A. Scirrhous carcinoma   B. Fibrocystic disease
    C. Duct papilloma   D. Paget's disease

Ans.	94. A	95. C	96. B	97. A	98. B	99. B
	100. A	101. C	102. C			

103. Which carcinoma breast is not invasive :
    A. Comedo carcinoma   B. Schirrhous carcinoma
    C. Lobular carcinoma   D. Paget's disease
104. The most favourable prognosis in breast carcinoma is associated with :
    A. Medullary carcinoma
    B. Scirrhous carcinoma
    C. Atrophic scirrhous carcinoma
    D. Duct carcinoma
    E. Invasive lobular carcinoma
105. A 50-year old post-menopausal woman has undergone modified radical mastectomy for a 4 cm sized T2 cancer breast. Examination of the axillary lymphnodes by the pathologist does not show any metastatic disease. Postoperative management of this patient would be :
    A. Radiotherapy
    B. Chemotherapy
    C. Tamoxifen
    D. Close monitoring and follow up
106. In inflammatory Ca breast with metastasis to axilla, treatment of choice is :
    A. Radical mastectomy + chemotherapy
    B. Radical mastectomy + radiotherapy
    C. Simple mastectomy + Radiotherapy
    D. Chemotherapy + Radio therapy
107. Most malignant type of carcinoma breast is :
    A. Paget's disease
    B. Anaplastic carcinoma
    C. Scirrhous's carcinoma
    D. Atrophic Scirrhous's carcinoma
    E. Mastitis carcinomatosa
108. Of the following pathological findings in the breast, which is least likely to be precancerous :
    A. Fibroadenoma   B. Intraductal papilloma
    C. Sclerosing adenosis   D. Lobular hyperplasia
    E. Cancer of one breast
109. The recurrence of carcinoma breast is indicated by enlargement of :
    A. Axillarylymph nodes   B. Cervical lymph nodes
    C. Dysphagia   D. Dypnoea

Ans.	103. A	104. A	105. D	106. B	107. E	108. A
	109. A					

110. A solitary breast mass is malignant if following are present except :
    A. Serous discharge   B. Gritty sensation
    C. Oedema of arm   D. Skin involvement.

111. Carcinoma of the breast 4 cm. in size fixed to the pectoralis muscle would qualify as :
    A. Stage I   B. State II
    C. Stage III   D. Stage IV

112. A distressing complication of radical mastectomy β is :
    A. Paralysis of the fifth finger of the hand
    B. Oedema of the arm
    C. Loss of sensation of the medial side of the arm
    D. Frequent skin infections of the hand on the affected side

113. A painless, hard swelling of breast in old woman is generally due to :
    A. Cancer   B. Calcified haematoma
    C. Fat necrosis   D. Fibroadenoma

114. Match List I (Clinical stage of breast cancer) with List II (Therapeutic option) and select the correct answer by using the codes given below the Lists:

List I		List II
A.	T1NoMo	1. Modified radical mastectomy + adjuvant chemotherapy
B.	T2N1Mo	2. Quadrantectomy + radiotherapy
C.	T4N2Mo	3. Palliative chemotherapy/Hormone therapy
D.	T4N2M1	4. Primary chemotherapy + adjuvant surgery

    Codes:

	a	b	c	d
A.	2	1	3	4
B.	1	2	4	3
C.	1	2	3	4
D.	2	1	4	3

115. Breast mass of 6 x 3 cm size with hard mobile ipsilateral axillary lymph node and ipsilateral supra clavicular lymph node, the staging is :
    A. $T_4N_2M_0$ B. $T_3N_2M_0$
    C. $T_3N_1M_1$ D. $T_4N_1M_1$

Ans.   110. A   111. C   112. B   113. B   114. D   115. C

116. Regarding moderately increased risk for Invasive Breast carcinoma which of the following conditions is true ?
    A. Sclerosing adenoma   B. Apocrine metaplasia
    C. Duct Ectasia   D. Atypical ductal hyperlasia
    E. Fibro adenoma
117. 4 cm breast nodule with ipsilatral mobile LN in axilla staging :
    A. $T_2N_1M_0$ B. $T_2N_2M_0$
    C. $T_1N_1M_0$ D. $T_3N_2M_1$
118. In which one of the following types of carcinoma of the breast, is a biopsy of the opposite breast advised ?
    A. Inflammatory carcinoma   B.Medullary carcinoma
    C. Lobular carcinoma   D. Scirrhous carcinoma
119. A 45 year old woman presents with hard and mobile lump in breast confirmatory investigation is :
    A. FNAC   B. USG
    C. Mammography   D. Excision biopsy
120. In a female patient of Breast Cancer with lung metastasis, the most common presenting symptoms is :
    A. Chronic cough   B. Hemoptysis
    C. No specific complaint   D. Dyspnoea
121. Worst prognosis in breast carcinoma is seen in :
    A. Colloid   B. Lobular
    C. Inflamatory   D. Papillary
122. After radical mastectomy there was injury to the long thoracic nerve. The integrity of the nerve can be tested at the bedside by asking the patient to?
    A. Shrug the shoulders
    B. Raise the arm above the head on the affected side
    C. Touch the opposite shoulder
    D. Lift a heavy object from the ground
123. All of the following are hormonal agents used against breast cancer except?
    A. Letrazole   B. Exemestrane
    C. Taxol   D. Tamoxifen
124. Which of the following microscopic features is typical of Paget's disease :
    A. Presence oflarge vaculoated cells
    B. Epidermal hypertrophy
    C. Subdermal round cell infiltration
    D. All of the above

Ans.	116. D	117. A	118. C	119. D	120. C	121. C
	122. B	123. C	124. D			

EYE & ENT

1. **The most frequently encountered malignant tumour of the nose and paranasal sinus :**
   A. Adenocarcinoma
   B. Basal cell carcinoma
   C. Squamous cell carcinoma
   D. Cylindroma
   E. Mixed tumour

2. **Maxillary sinus carcinoma may be caused by :**
   A. Aniline dye   B. Auramine
   C. Petroleum jelly   D. Irradiation

3. **In malignancies of nasal cavities the chief symptoms is :**
   A. Repeated unilateral epistaxis
   B. Continuous purulent and sanguineous discharge
   C. Headache
   D. Broadening of nasal bones

4. **Virus induced carcinoma is :**
   A. Ca nasal cavity   B. Ca maxillary sinus
   C. Nasopharyngeal Ca   D. Ca larynx

5. **Angiofibroma responds to which of the following modalities of treatment :**
   A. Surgery   B. Radiotherapy
   C. Hormonal therapy   D. Immunotherapy

6. **Best treatment of early nasopharyngeal carcinoma is :**
   A. Surgery   B. Radiotherapy
   C. Surgery+Rdiotherapy D. Drugs

7. **Indication of radiotherapy in nasopharyngeal angiofibroma is invasion of :**
   A. Orbit   B. Middle cranial fossa
   C. Paranasal sinuses   D. Palate

8. **Treatment of maxillary antral carcinoma (T3 No) is :**
   A. Only surgery
   B. Surgery and radiotherapy
   C. Chemotherapy and radiotherapy
   D. Radiotherapy only

Ans.	1. C	2. D	3. A	4. C	5. A	6. B
	7. B	8. B				

9. Malignant tumours are most common in which of the following sinuses ?
    A. Sphenoidal sinus   B. Frontal sinus
    C. Ethmoidal sinuses   D. Maxillary sinus
10. Most common site of osteoma is :
    A. Frontal sinus   B. Maxillary sinus
    C. Sphenoidal sinus   D. Nasopharynx
11. Malignant tumour arising from paranasal sinuses is commonly seen in :
    A. Frontal   B. Ethmodal
    C. Maxillary   D. Sphenoid
12. True about inverted papilloma is following except :
    A. Fragile
    B. Nasal obstruction
    C. Carcinoma develops
    D. Treated by adequate local excision
13. Fibroma of the nasopharynx :
    A. Is most common in young boys
    B. May extend into cranial fossa
    C. Bleeds extensively at biopsy
    D. All of the above
14. Nasopharyngeal angiofibroma is seen in :
    A. Elderly people
    B. Infants
    C. Adolescents males
    D. Adolescents females
15. The ethmoidal sinus carcinoma is seen in :
    A. Chimney smokers   B. Dye makers
    C. Watch makers   D. Cotton industry
16. Carcinoma of maxillary antrum most often presents with :
    A. Unilateral nasal obstruction
    B. Chek or palate swelling
    C. Epistaxis
    D. Trismus
    E. Cervical lymph nodes
17. Maxillary carcinoma is associated with :
    A. Wood dust   B. Betelnut chewing
    C. EBV   D. None

Ans.	9. D	10. A	11. C	12. C	13. D	14. C
	15. A	16. A	17. A			

18. **Secondary deposits from the maxillary antrum is seen in region :**
    A. Upper deep cervical   B. Lower deep cervical
    C. Supra clavicular   D. Submandibular

19. **Nasopharyngeal carcinoma commonly presents as :**
    A. Recurrent epistaxis   B. Bilateral neck mass
    C. Frontal sinusitis   D. Ocular palsy

20. **Wrong about nasal fibroangioma is :**
    A. Epistaxis   B. May regress with age
    C. Metastasis   D. Common in chidren

21. **Nasopharyngeal carcinoma is common in :**
    A. Caucasians   B. Neogroes
    C. Europeans   D. None of the above

22. **Which of the following anatomical type of Carcinoma of maxillary sinus is least harmful :**
    A. Posterior superior medial
    B. Posterior superior lateral
    C. Anterior inferior medial
    D. Anterior inferior lateral

23. **HLA in nasopharyngeal carcinoma is :**
    A. A3   B. DW3
    C. B27   D. None of the above

24. **Hairy palpoidal mass in nasopharynx may by :**
    A. Nasopharyngeal angiofibroma
    B. Ganiopharyngioma
    C. Chordoma
    D. Dermoid cyst

25. **Bleeding nasal tumor is given the name :**
    A. Polyp   B. Papilloma
    C. Rhinoscleroma   D. Angiofibroma

26. **Angiofibroma bleeds excessively because :**
    A. It lacks a capsule
    B. Vessels lack a contractile component
    C. It has multiple sites of origin
    D. All of the above

27. **A child presented with history of unilateral purulent nasal discharge with occasional bloody discharge from the same side. The diagnosis is:**
    A. Antrachoanal polyp   B. Foreign body
    C. Angiofibroma   D. Rhinosporidiosis

Ans.	18. A	19. A	20. C	21. D	22. C	23. D
	24. A	25. D	26. B	27. C		

28. The earliest symptom in retinoblastoma is :
    A. Strabismus
    B. Poor vision
    C. Proptosis
    D. Leucokoria (cat's eye reflex)

29. The following about retinoblastoma is true except :
    A. Autosomal dominant
    B. Treatment is enculeation
    C. Radiotherapy is also given
    D. Eviseration is the treatment

30. Most common second malignancy in patients with Familial Retinoblastoma is:
    A Teratoma.   B   Medullary carcinoma.
    C Osteosarcoma.   D   Malignant melanoma.

31. Most common tumor of lid is :
    A. Basal cell Ca
    B. Malignant melanoma
    C. Angle closure glaucoma
    D. Cataract

32. The commonest tumour of the lacrimal gland is :
    A. Adenoma
    B. Carcinoma
    C. Granuloma
    D. Benign mixed tumour
    E. Pleomorphic Adenocarcinoma

33. Frontal lobe lesions may cause all of the following except :
    A. Exophthalmos
    B. Unilateral lowering of visual acuity
    C. Superior quadrantic field defect
    D. Changes in corneal reflex
    E. Gaze-paretic nystagmus to opposite site

34. The commonest intra-ocular tumour in children is :
    A. Malignant melanoma
    B. Retinoblastoma
    C. Teratoid medulloepithelioma
    D. Diktyoma

35. Gradual enlargement of optic canal is seen in :
    A. Retinoblastoma   B.   Neurofibromatasis
    C. Haemangioma   D.   Meningioma

Ans.	28. D	29. D	30. C	31. A	32. E	33. C
	34. B	35. D				

36. Foster Kennedy syndrome is seen in all except :
    A. Frontal meningioma
    B. Frontal lobe glioma
    C. Optic glioma
    D. Meningioma of olfactory tract
    E. Medulloblastoma in cerebellum

37. The mother of a one and a half year old child gives history of a while reflex from one eye for the past 1 month. On computed tomography scan of the orbit there is calcification seen within the globe. The most likely diagnosis is :
    A. Congenital cataract
    B. Retinoblastoma
    C. Endophthalmitis
    D. Coats disease

38. The most frequent symptom of cancer of nasopharynx is :
    A. Mass in the neck   B. Blocked nose
    C. Diplopia   D. Epistaxis

39. The predisposing factor in hypopharyngeal cancer is :
    A. Vocal cord infection
    B. Plummer vinson's syndrome
    C. Chronic tonsillitis
    D. Leucoplakia of cord

40. The commonest symptoms of nasopharyngeal carcinoma (fossa of Rosenmuller) is :
    A. Epistaxis   B. Neck mass
    C. Nasal block   D. Deafness
    E. Aural fullness.

41. In postcricoid carcinoma, the treatment of choice is :
    A. Total larynegectomy
    B. Total laryngectomy + Pharyngectomy
    C. b+radiotherapy
    D. Only radiotherapy

42. In cancer of postcricoid region, the treatment of choice is :
    A. Chemotherapy   B. Surgery
    C. Radiotherapy   D. b+c

43. Which is true of nasopharyngeal carcinoma :
    A. Good prognosis   B. Can be cured by surgery
    C. Spread to lymph nodes   D. Etiology is unknown

Ans.	36. E	37. B	38. A	39. B	40. E	41. C
	42. D	43. C				

44. Carcinoma of palate has folowing features except :
A. Adeno carcinoma
B. Slow growing
C. Presents with pain
D. Bilateral lympahtic spread

45. Best diagnosis of Nasopharyngeal angiofibroma is :
A. Angiography   B. Contrast enhanced CT
C. MRI   D. X-ray

46. Which is true of nasopharyngeal carinoma :
A. Good prognosis   B. Can be cured by surgery
C. Spread to lymph nodes D. Etiology is unknown

47. Features of firboangioma of the nasopharynx include :
A. It is a highly destructive B. It is a benign tumour
C. Never metastasises   D. It causes a 'frog facies'
E. All of the above

48. In pyriform fossa carcinoma, prognosis is poor because :
A. Lymph nodes are not involved
B. Present early
C. Metastasis frequent
D. Radioresistant

49. Lateral retropharyngeal lymph node of Ranvier are involved in carcinoma of :
A. Glottis   B. Oropharynx
C. Oesophagus   D. Nasopharynx

50. Nasopharyngeal carcinoma arises from :
A. Lat. wall of nose
B. Medial wall of nose
C. Sphenopalatine foramen
D. Maxillary antrum

51. Treatment of choice for T carcinoma of nasopharynx is :
A. Surgery
B. Radiotherapy
C. Chemotherapy
D. Surgery + Post Operative Radiotherapy

52. Vocal nodules are commonly present on vocal cords at :
A. Anterior end
B. Posterior end
C. At junction of anterior third and posterior 2/3 rd
D. At the mid level
E. At the junction of anterior 2/3rd and   posterior 1/3rd

Ans.	44. B	45. B	46. C	47. E	48. C	49. D
	50. C	51. B	52. C			

53. **Carcinoma larynx with no neck secondaries is treated by :**
    A. Laryngectomy
    B. Laryngectomy and radical neck dissection
    C. Radiation
    D. Radiation and laryngectomy

54. **Which variety of laryngeal carcinoma has the best prognosis ?**
    A. Laryngopharynx   B. Glottic (Vocal cord)
    C. Subglottic   D. Supraglottic

55. **Most useful procedure for the diagnosis of carcinoma larynx is :**
    A. X-ray of soft tissue neck
    B. Indirect laryngoscopy
    C. Direct laryngoscopy
    D. Laryngogram

56. **Treatment of choice in subglottic carcinoma is :**
    A. Total laryngectomy   B. Partial laryngectomy
    C. Chemotherapy   D. Radiotherapy

57. **Stridor is a manifestation of :**
    A. Early glottic cancer   B. Bilateral cord paralysis
    C. Leukoplakia   D. Vocal cord nodules

58. **Staging of 6 cm growth in cheek with bila-teral mobile lymph nodes :**
    A. T3N   B. T4N2
    C. T4N3   D. T3N3

59. **Treatment of multiple papilloma of the larynx is :**
    A. Excision with laser   B. Excision with cautery
    C. Chemotherapy   D. Hormonal therapy

60. **Treatment of choice for stage I laryngeal carcinoma is :**
    A. Resection of vocal cord
    B. Radiotherapy
    C. Striping of vocal cord
    D. Laryngectomy

61. **True about Glottic tumor is :**
    A. Lymphatic spread common
    B. Better prognosis than subglottic type
    C. Most common site is post commisure
    D. Sticky sensation on throat commonest symptom

62. **Chondroma is commonest in ———— cartilage :**
    A. Arytenoids   B. Cricoid
    C. Thyroid   D. Epiglottis

Ans.	53. C	54. B	55. C	56. A	57. B	58. A
	59. A	60. B	61. B	62. B		

63. **Regarding multiple papillomas in the larynx which of the following statements are correct :**
   A. Common in infants and children
   B. Viral in origin
   C. Vocal cords usual site
   D. Treatment is removal by direct laryngoscopy
   E. All are correct

64. **Granuloma of the vocal cords is mostly due to :**
   A. Intubation   B.   Syphilis
   C. Malignancy   D.   Vocal abuse

65. **Precancerous condition of the larynx include all except :**
   A. Syphilis   B.   Papilloma
   C. Leukoplakia   D.   None of the above

66. **A laryngeal polyp :**
   A. Usually occurs on the anterior two thirds of the vocal cords
   B. Is covered by pseudostratified ciliated celumnar epithelium
   C. Both
   D. Neither

67. **Papilloma in larynx is characterized by all except :**
   A. Viral in origin
   B. Multiple
   C. Best treated by radiotherapy
   D. Initial treatment is local removal
   E. Most common laryngeal tumours in children

68. **The treatment of choice in Stage II glottic carcinoma is :**
   A. Radiotherapy   B.   Surgery
   C. Chemotherapy   D.   Surgery + Chemotherapy

69. **Earliest symptom of Carcinoma vocal cord is : Delhi 1988**
   A. Hoarseness   B.   Stridor
   C. Pain   D.   Dysphagia

70. **Juvenile Multiple laryngeal Papilloma is caused by :**
   A. Bacteria   B.   Virus
   C. Neoplastic   D.   None of the above

71. **Childhood papilloma of larynx has —— aetiology :**
   A. Viral   B.   Bacterial
   C. Chlamydia   D.   Fungus

72. **Carcinoma in situ of larynx is treated by :**
   A. Radiotherapy   B.   Stripping
   C. Partial laryngectomy   D.   Total laryngectomy

Ans.	63. E	64. A	65. A	66. A	67. C	68. A
	69. A	70. B	71. A	72. B		

73. **Laryngeal cancers are mostly :**
    A. Squmous cell carcinomas
    B. Adenocarcinomas
    C. Sarcomas
    D. Transitional cell carcinoma

74. **Treatment of Glottic carcinoma is :**
    A. Radiotherapy   B. Chemotherapy
    C. Surgery   D. Radiotherapy + Surgery

75. **Which is not a feature of childhood laryngeal papilloma ?**
    A. Multiple   B. Viral origin
    C. Permalignant   D. Recurrent

76. **Commonest site of carcinoma larynx in females is :**
    A. Vocal cord   B. Pyryform fossa
    C. Posterior cricoid   D. False cord

77. **Good prognosis in glottic carcinoma is because of :**
    A. Rapid spread   B. No lymphatics
    C. Apnoea   D. No prominent symptoms

78. **Singer's nodule is mostly seen at :**
    A. Junction of ant 2/3 and post 1/3 vocal cords
    B. Junction of ant 1/3 & post 2/3 vocal cords
    C. Middle of ant 1/3 & 2/3 vocal cords
    D. Any where

79. **A person is given radiotherapy to superior sulcus lung tumor, develops horseness of voice probable cause is :**
    A. Invasion of nerve by tumor
    B. Damage to larynx byradiation
    C. Secondaries into vocal cord
    D. Ca larynx due to radiation

80. **Commonest neoplasm in vocal cord in pediatric age group :**
    A. Solitary papilloma   B. Multiple papilloma
    C. Carcinoma   D. Fibroma

81. **A 55-year-old smoker presents with complaints of hemoptysis. On bronchoscopic examiantion, there was a lesion in the distal trachea which was growing in to the lumen. Which of the following is the most probabale diagnosis :**
    A. Squamous cell carcinoma
    B. Adenoid cystic carcinoma
    C. Squamous papilloma
    D. Muco epidermoid carcinoma

82. **Most radiosensitive tumour of the following is :**
    A. Supraglottic ca   B. Ca glottis
    C. Ca nasopharynx   D. Subglottic ca

Ans.	73. A	74. A	75. C	76. C	77. B	78. B
	79. A	80. B	81. A	82. B		

83. The treatment of choice of a glottic cancer with stage $T_1N_0M_0$ is :
   A. Brachytherapy
   B. External beam radiotherapy
   C. Laryngectomy
   D. Chemotherapy

84. A chronic smoker with history of hoarseness was found on examination to have keratosis of the larynx. All the following are possible treatment modalities except :
   A. Laser
   B. Radiotherapy
   C. Stripping of the vocal cor
   D. Partial laryngectomy

85. Hoarsness secondary to bronchogenic carcinoma is usually due to extension of the tumour into :
   A. Vocal cord
   B. Superior laryngeal nerve
   C. Left recurrent laryngeal nerve
   D. Right vagus nerve

86. Vocal cord paralysis on the left side in an elderly person is commonly with :
   A. Bronchogenic carcinoma
   B. Aneurysm of carotid artery
   C. Malignancy neck
   D. Malignancy of lower jaw

87. The most common and earliest manifestation of carcinoma of the glottis is :
   A. Hoarseness   B. Haemoptysis
   C. Cervical lymph nodes   D. Stridor

88. Areas of carcinoma of oral mucosa can be identified by staining with :
   A. 1% zinc chloride   B. 2% silver nitrate
   C. Gentian violet   D. 2% toluidine blue
   E. 10% Congro red

89. In carcinoma of tip of tongue, lymph nodes not involved are :
   A. Jugulodiagastric   B. Retropharyngeal
   C. Submandibular   D. None of the above

90. Which of the following is a premalignant condition?
   A. Aphthous stomatitis   B. Chronic glossitis
   C. Hypertrophic glossitis D. Submucous fibrosis

Ans.	83. B	84. A	85. C	86. A	87. A	88. D
	89. B	90. D				

91. **Feature of the glomus jugulare tumour may include all except :**
    A. Females are commonly affected
    B. Pulsating tinnitus
    C. Otalgia
    D. It is disease of infancy

92. **Hyposthesia of the posterior aspect of the external auditory canal may be an early sign of :**
    A. Trigeminal neuralgia
    B. Costen's syndrome
    C. Lateral sinus thrombosis
    D. Multiple sclerosis
    E. Acoustic neuroma

93. **Carcinoma of the pinna :**
    A. A basal cell carcinoma
    B. Best treated by radiotherapy
    C. May require the ear to be cut off
    D. All of the above

94. **Acoustic neuroma commonly affects the :**
    A. 5th cranial nerve   B. 6th cranial nerve
    C. 7th cranial nerve   D. 8th cranial nerve

95. **Acoustic neuroma commonly affects which nerve ?**
    A. V   B. VI
    C. VII   D. VIII

96. **In Acoustic neuroma, most common involvement is :**
    A. Cochlear nuclei
    B. Supravestibular nuclei
    C. Inferior vestibular nuclei
    D. Trigeminal nuclei

97. **In acoustic neuroma, audiometric change occurs first at :**
    A. 1000 Hz   B. 2000 Hz
    C. 3000 Hz   D. 4000 Hz

98. **The usually location of glomus jugulare tumour is :**
    A. Epitympanum   B. Hypotympanum
    C. Mastoid tip cells   D. Promontory
    E. Internal auditory meatus

99. **The treatment of choice of glomus jugulare tumour is :**
    A. Watchful waiting   B. Surgical removal
    C. Irradiation   D. Chemotherapy

100. **The earliest symptom of acoustic neuroma is :**
    A. Headache   B. Vertigo
    C. Hearing loss   D. Corneal anaesthesia
    E. Facial weakness

Ans.	91. D	92. E	93. C	94. D	95. D	96. B
	97. D	98. B	99. B	100. C		

101. Dangerous variety of neurofibroma is :
   A. Acoustic neuroma
   B. Pachy neurofibroma
   C. Generalised neurofibroma
   D. None

102. Commonest site of tumour in ear is :
   A. Auricle   B. Middle ear
   C. Inner ear   D. None

103. Acoustic neuroma causes :
   A. Cochlear deafness   B. Retrocochlear deafness
   C. Conductive deafness   D. Any of the above

104. Consider the following statements :
   Acoustic neuroma
   1. Is usually bilaterial
   2. Does not alter CSF biochemistry
   3. May cause vertigo
   4. Gives rise to pyramidal lesion
   Which of the above statements are correct ?
   A. 1,.2 and 3   B. 2, and 3
   C. 3 and 4   D. 1 and 4

105. True statement about glomus jugulare tumor is :
   A. Common in males
   B. May involve V to VII cranial nerves
   C. Arises from promontary of middle ear
   D. Benign non-encapsulated vascular tumor

106. In a patient with acoustic neuroma all are seen except :
   A. Facial nerve may be involved
   B. Tinnitus is present
   C. Deafness
   D. Acute episodes of vertigo occur

107. A patient is suspected to have vestibular shwanomma. The investigation of choice for its diagnosis is :
   A. Contrast enhanced CT scan
   B. Gadolinium enhanced MRI
   C. SPECT
   D. PET scan

Ans.	101. A	102. A	103. A	104. C	105. D	106. A
	107. A					

THERAPEUTICS

1. **6-Mercaptopurine potentiates action of :**
   A. Cyclophosphamide   B. Allopurinol
   C. Methotrexate   D. 5-FU

2. **Example of an immunostimulant drug is :**
   A. Cyclosporine
   B. Antilymphocytic globulin (ALG)
   C. Drug induced erythematosus
   D. Methyldopa induced hemolytic anemia

3. **Not given intrathecally :**
   A. Methotrexate   B. Taxol
   C. 5FU   D. Cyclophosphamide

4. **Which of the following is not an alkylating agent :**
   A. Cytarbine   B. Chlorambucil
   C. Cyclophosphamide   D. Thiotepa

5. **Which cytotoxic drug inhibits cellular division in mitosis (i.e. metaphase arrest) :**
   A. Vincristine   B. 5-FU
   C. Methotrexate   D. Cyclophosphamide

6. **5-FU is the chemotherapeutic drug of choice in the following solid tumors except :**
   A. Pancreas   B. Breast
   C. Colon   D. Stomach

7. **Chemotherapeutic agent used in Wilm's tumor is :**
   A. Methotrexate   B. Cyclophosphamide
   C. 5-FU   D. Actinomycin D

8. **Leukoencephalopathy is seen with use of :**
   A. Vincristine   B. Cyclophosphamide
   C. Methotrexate   D. 5-FU

9. **Following are true about cyclophosphamide except :**
   A. Orally ineffective
   B. Useful in Ca breast
   C. Cause haemorrhagic cystitis
   D. Potent immunosuppressent

10. **A example of pyrimidine antagonist is :**
    A. Busulfan   B. Flurorouracil
    C. Cyclophosphamide   D. Mercaptopurine

Ans.	1. B	2. B	3. B	4. A	5. A	6. A
	7. D	8. C	9. A	10. B		

11. Which is not an alkylating agent :
    A. Chlorambucil   B. Cyclophosphamide
    C. Thiotepa   D. 6- mercaptopurine
12. Actinomycin D acts on :
    A. Tranduction   B. Translation
    C. Transcription   D. Translocation
13. Which of the following anti-cancer drugs does not cause bone marrow suppression?
    A. Bleomycin   B. Cyclophosphamide
    C. Methotrexate   D. Vinblastin
14. Which among the following is not an immuno-supressant :
    A. Cyclosporine   B. Cromolyn glycate
    C. Azathioprine   D. None
15. Which antimalignancy drug is most nephrotoxic :
    A. Vincristine   B. Cyclophosphamide
    C. Cisplatinum   D. Methotrexate
    E. 5-FU
16. Melphalan is drug of choice in :
    A. Malignant melanoma B. Neuroblastoma
    C. Retinoblastoma   D. Hypernephroma
17. Drug acting on mitotic phase of cell cycle is :
    A. Methotrexate   B. 5-FU
    C. Vincristine   D. Procarbazine
18. Treatment of acute lymphoblastic leukemia in child with CNS manifestations is :
    A. Intrathecal methotrexate
    B. Vincristine and prednisolone
    C. Intrathecal vincristine
    D. Intrathecal steroids and vincristine
19. Which is not an alkylating agent :
    A. Methotrexate   B. Melphalan
    C. Chlorambucil   D. Cyclophosphamide
W.20. Radiation recall phenomenon is seen with :
    A. Doxrubicin   B. Cis-Platinum
    C. Cyclophosphamide D. Adriamycin
21. In Cisplatinum induced emesis drug of choice is :
    A. Ondasterone   B. Metaclopramide
    C. Domperidone   D. Octreotide
22. The commonest side effect of 5-Fluorouracil is :
    A. Bone marrow depression
    B. Gastrointestinal tract ulceration

Ans.	11. D	12. C	13. B	14. D	15. C	16. A
	17. C	18. A	19. A	20. NONE	21. A	22. B

C. Hypersensitivity reaction
D. Diarrhoea

23. **In hairy cell leukemia, treatment of choice is :**
    A. Alkylating agent   B. Corticosteroid
    C. Splenectomy   D. Pentostatin

24. **Drug of choice in breast cancer :**
    A. Melphalan   B. Fluorouracil
    C. Cyclophosphamide   D. Methotrexate

25. **The dose of 6—mercaptopurine requires reduction with intake of :**
    A. Allopurinol   B. Folic acid
    C. Azathioprine   D. Vitamin B12

26. **Which of the following antineoplastic agents does not require biotransformation to exert its cytotoxic action ?**

    A. 5-fluorouracil   B. Cytarabine
    C. Thioguanine   D. 6-mercaptopurin

27. **Ifosfamide belongs to :**
    A. Alkylating agents   B. Antimetabolites
    C. Antibiotics   D. None of the above

28. **Drug useful in chronic myeloid leukaemia :**
    A. Chlorambacil   B. Busulphan
    C. Melphalan   D. Vincristine

29. **Ifosfamide is a congener of :**
    A. Mustine HCl   B. Adriamycin
    C. Cyclophosphamide   D. Methotrexate

30. **Mode of action of Actiomycin D is to prevent :**
    A. RNA elongation   B. DNA synthesis
    C. DNA elongation   D. None of the above

31. **To achieve pleurodesmosis in malignant pleural effusion, the drug used is :**
    A. Polymyxin B   B. Chlormycetin
    C. 1% Betadine   D. Tetracycline

32. **Drug of choice in acute lymphatic leukaemia is :**
    A. Mercaptopurine
    B. Cyclophosphamide
    C. Methotrexate
    D. Vincristine+Predinisolone

33. **Drug of choice in multiple myeloma is :**
    A. Prednisolone   B. Cyclophosphamide
    C. Melphalan   D. Mechlorethamin

Ans.	23. D	24. C	25. A	26. D	27. A	28. B
	29. C	30. A	31. D	32. D	33. C	

34. Successful treatment with single drug in Hodgkin's disease has been seen with :
   A. Procarbarine   B. Mithramycin
   C. Mechlorethamine   D. Radio phosphorus

35. Dose of 6-mercaptopurine requires reduction with :
   A. Allopurinol   B. Thiazide
   C. Methotrexate   D. Spironolactone

36. Mycosis fungoides is best treated by :
   A. 5-FU cream   B. Election beam therapy
   C. Surgery   D. I/V Adriamycin

37. Which of the following does not cause bone marrow suppression :
   A. Cisplatin   B. Daunorubicin
   C. Vincristine   D. Cyclophosphamide

38. Which of the following crosses blood brain barrier :
   A. Cyclophospamide   B. Ciaplatin
   C. 5-FU   D. Procarbazine

39. Following drugs are known immuno suppressive agents except :
   A. Prednisolone   B. Cephalosporin
   C. Azathioprine   D. Cyclosporin A

40. Which is an immune stimulant :
   A. Vidarabine   B. Methimazole
   C. Levamisole   D. Zudovidine

41. All of the following are Dihydrofolate reductase inhibitor except ;
   A. Methotrexate   B. Pyrimethamine
   C. Pentamidine   D. Cytosine arabinoside

42. Busulfan toxicity does not include :
   A. Hyperpigmentation   B. Toxic carditis
   C. Hyperuricemia   D. Pulmonary fibrosis

43. L-asparaginase is used in treatment of :
   A. AML   B. CML
   C. ALL   D. CLL

44. Methotrexate acts by :
   A. Folic acid antagonism   B. Purine antagonism
   C. Pyramidine antagonism   D. All of the above

45. 5-FU is not used in ———— cancer :
   A. Liver   B. Stomach
   C. Mycosis fungoides   D. Breast

46. Following are sideeffects of chemotherapeutic agents except :
   A. Dermatitis   B. Teratogenicity
   C. BM suppression   D. Hypertension

Ans.	34. C	35. A	36. B	37. A	38. D	39. A
	40. C	41. C	42. B	43. C	44. A	45. C
	46. D					

47. **Cyclophosphamide is used in following except :**
   A. Burkitt's lymphoma   B. Hodgkin's lymphoma
   C. Choriocarcinoma   D. Ovarian carcinoma

48. **Both phase anti-cancer drugs are following except :**
   A. Vincristine   B. 5-FU
   C. Nitrogen mustard   D. L-Asparaginase

49. **Chlorambucil is a :**
   A. Pyramidine analog   B. Piperdine analog
   C. Folic acid analog   D. Alkylating agent

50. **Choriocarcinoma with jaundice—treatment of choice :**
   A. Actinomycin-D   B. Methotrexate
   C. 5-MC   D. Busulphan

51. **Cyclophosphamide induced cystitis is prevented by :**
   A. Allopurinol   B. Acetyl cysteine
   C. Necetral soap water   D. Phenozopyridine

52. **Most common regime used in Ca breast is :**
   A. CMF   B. CAV
   C. HOP   D. PEB

53. **MOPP regime includes :**
   A. N2 mustard, Adriamycin, Prednisolone, Procarbazine
   B. Cyclophosphamide, Adriamycin, Prednisolone, Procarbazine
   C. Mitoxantrene, Adriamycin, Prednisolone, Procarbazine
   D. Mechlorethamine, Vincristine, Adriamycin, Prednisolone, Procarbazine

54. **Cyclosporine acts on :**
   A. B-lymphocytes   B. T-lymphocytes
   C. Mitochondria   D. Ribosomes

55. **Cirrhosis of liver is caused by :**
   A. Mitomycin   B. Cyclophosphamide
   C. Methotrexate   D. 6-thioguanine

56. **Tetra hydro folate inhibitor, not true is :**
   A. Methotrexate   B. Pyrimethamine
   C. Pentamidine   D. Cytosine Arabinose

57. **Drug of choice in ALL is :**
   A. 6-Mercaptopurine   B. Vincristine
   C. L-asparaginase   D. Methotrexate

58. **Drug which acts very fastly than any other in the following to ↓ the serum calcium :**
   A. Bleomycin   B. Mithramycin
   C. Calcitonin   D. Insulin

Ans.	47. C	48. A	49. D	50. A	51. B	52. A
	53. D	54. A	55. C	56. D	57. B	58. B

59. **Imipenem combined with cilastatin is more useful because :**
    A. It inhibits the metabolism of imipenem
    B. It increases more bioavailability of the drug
    C. It increases the synthesis of the imipenem
    D. It causes reversible inhibition of dihydropeptidase

60. **Methotrexate is most useful in :**
    A. Abruptio placentae   B. Ectopic pregnancy
    C. Placenta accreta   D. Trophoblastic disease

61. **An antifolate which is an immunosuppressant is :**
    A. Pyrimethamine   B. 5 FU
    C. Cyclophosphamide   D. Methotrexate

62. **Mesna is given with cyclophosphamide because :**
    A. Decreases toxicity of cyclophosphamide on bladder
    B. It increases effectiveness of cyclophosphamide
    C. It increases metabolism of cyclophosphamide
    D. It prevents vomiting

63. **Match List I (Immunosuppressive drugs) with List II (Side effects) and select the correct answer using the codes given below the lists :**

    List I   List II
    A. Azathioprine   1. Cushinoid appearance
    B. Steroid   2. Leukopenia and hepatotoxicity
    C. Cyclosporine   3. Pulmonary oedema and CNS disturbance
    D. OKT3   4. Nephrotoxicity

    Codes :

	A	B	C	D
A.	2	1	4	3
B.	1	2	3	4
C.	2	1	3	4
D.	1	2	4	3

64. **Radioisotope I^{131} undergoes 99% decay in:**
    A. 36 days   B. 26 days
    C. 46 days   D. 56 days

65. **In kidney, Cisplain causes :**
    A. Direct toxicity
    B. Glomerular damage
    C. Tubular damage
    D. Bowman's capsule damage

Ans.	59.	60. D	61. D	62. A	63. C	64. D
	65. A					

66. **Which of the following inhibits transcription :**
   A. 5-Flurouracil
   B. Rifamycin
   C. Cyclosporine
   D. Cyclophosphamide

67. **A patient with Hodgkin's lymphoma is having a single cervical lymphnode. Biopsy showed lymphocyte predominant variant. Which of the following is the treatment of choice :**
   A. Chemotherapy with Radiotherapy
   B. Chemotherapy only
   C. Radiotherapy only
   D. No treatment needed

68. **All of the following are correct about alkylating agent except :**
   A. Folinic acid completely terminates the action of methotrexate
   B. Melphalan may cause pancreatitis
   C. Mesna inactivates the vesicotoxic metabolites of cyclophos-phamide
   D. Ifosfamide causes less alopecia than cyclophos-phamide

69. **The drug not used in prostatic carcinoma :**
   A. Finasteride
   B. Diethyl stilbestrol
   C. Testosteron
   D. Flutamide

70. **All the following are true are true about paclitaxel except :**
   A. It acts on the mitotic phase
   B. Improves microtubule formation
   C. Oral Bioavailability is very high
   D. Extensively metabolized by liver

71. **Gemicitabine is effective in cancers of the :**
   A. Head and neck
   B. Pancreas
   C. Lung
   D. Soft tissue sarcoma

72. **After load intracavitory radiation is used in :**
   A. Carcinoma Cervix
   B. Carcinoma of colon
   C. Amoebiasis
   D. Crohn's disease

73. **Most radiosensitive lung cancer is :**
   A. Adenocarcinoma
   B. Squamous cell carcinoma
   C. Anaplastic carcinoma
   D. Giant cell carcinoma

74. **Most sensitive test for metastaic deposit is :**
   A. Isotope scan
   B. CT scan
   C. Skeletal survey
   D. Epilepsy
   E. Vascular lesions

75. **Drug used for Ca oesophagus is :**
   A. Cisplatin
   B. Adriamycin
   C. Cyclosporin
   D. Actinomycin D

Ans.	66. C	67. C	68. A	69. C	70. C	71. B
	72. A	73. B	74. A	75. A		

76. The following tumours respond very well to irradia-tion therapy except :
    A. Squamous cell carcinoma
    B. Seminoma
    C. Brain tumour
    D. Soft tissue sarcoma

77. Most radiosensitive cancer among the following is :
    A. Basal cell Ca skin
    B. Squamous cell Ca Cx
    C. Small cell Ca lung
    D. Hepatocellular carcinoma

78. Radiation during childhood can cause :
    A. Lymphoma
    B. Papillary Ca. Thyroid
    C. Ca stomach
    D. Laryngeal Ca.

79. Chemotherapeutic agent used in Wilim's tumor is :
    A. Methotrexate
    B. Cyclophosphamide
    C. 5FU
    D. Actinomycin D

80. UV rays cause :
    A. Deletion of pyramidines
    B. Substitution of purine for pyrimidine
    C. Cross linking of purine with pyrimidine
    D. Dimerisation of pyrimidine

81. Commonest post irriadiation carcinoma of thyroid is :
    A. Papillary
    B. Follicular
    C. Medullary
    D. Anaplastic

82. Treatment by radiotherapy is most frequently indicated in carcinoma of :
    A. Ovary
    B. Lung
    C. Cervix
    D. Thyroid

83. The drug of choice for chemotherapy of retinoblastoma is :
    A. Vincristine
    B. Nitrogen mustard
    C. 5-fluorouracil (5FU)
    D. Triethylene melamine (TEM)

84. Oto-toxicity and nephrotoxicity are frequently encountered following therapy with :
    A. 5-F.U
    B. Endoxan
    C. Bleomycin
    D. Cis-Plantinum

85. 5-Fluoro-uracil is used in treatment of following cancers except :
    A. Breast
    B. Stomach
    C. Liver
    D. Mycosis fungoides

Ans.	76. D	77. B	78. B	79. D	80. D	81. A
	82. C	83. A	84. D	85. D		

86. Testicular tumour which responds best to radiation is :
    A. Teratoma
    B. Seminoma
    C. Embryonal cell carcinoma
    D. None of the above

87. The utility of adjuvant radiotherapy in the treatment of tumours is limited by all the following considerations except :
    A. Injury to normal tissues
    B. Oncogenic potential of treatment
    C. Activation of T lymphocytes
    D. Systemic subclinical disease

88. Radiotherapy is curable in :
    A. Ewing's tumour
    B. Osteosarcoma
    C. Rhabdomyosarcoma
    D. Squamous cell carcinoma of mouth

89. Which of the following malignant tumours is extemely resistant to radiation?
    A. Embryonal carcinoma   B. Fibrosarcoma
    C. Lymphosarcoma   D. Squamous cell carcinoma

90. Radio therapy is not used in :
    A. Ca oesophagus   B. Ca cervix
    C. Ca stomach   D. Brain tumour

91. Mantle radiation is given in :
    A. Hodgkin's lymphoma   B. Ca cervix
    C. Ca thyroid   D. Ca ovary

92. Commonest cancer treated by radiotherapy in India :
    A. CA Rectum   B. CA Cervix
    C. CA Liver   D. CA Stomach

93. Most radiosensitive sarcoma is :
    A. Liposarcoma   B. Fibrosarcoma
    C. Chondrosarcoma   D. Ewings sarcoma

94. In which malignancy postoperative radiotherapy is minimally used?
    A. Head and neck   B. Stomach
    C. Colon   D. Soft tissue sarcomas

95. Scintigraphy is used to demonstrate tumor in the :
    A. Breast   B. Stomach
    C. Rectum   D. Vertebral column
    E. Kidney

Ans.	86. B	87. C	88. A	89. A	90. C	91. A
	92. B	93. D	94. B	95. D		

96. Excretory urography should be cautiously performed in case of :
    A. Leukaemia   B. Neuroblastoma
    C. Bone secondaries   D. Multiple myeloma
97. Lymphangiography is useful in :
    A. Lymphomas   B. Gynaecological
    C. Testicular tumours   D. All of the above
98. In head and neck cancer patients, good oral hygiene is essential during radiotherapy :
    A. True
    B. Only during chemotherapy
    C. Only during surgery
    D. Combination treatment with chemotherapy and surgery

MISCELLANEOUS

1. **Appropriate initial treatment of breast carcinoma in a young girl is :**
   A. Adequate local excision
   B. Radical mastectamy
   C. Chemotherapy
   D. Radiotherapy

2. **The risks of developing breast carcinoma for daughters and sisters of women with Ca breast are —— respectively :**
   A. 10-28%, 7-14%   B. 30-40%, 15-30%
   C. 30-40%, 20-30%   D. 40-50%, 30-40%

3. **Following tumors metastasises to breast except :**
   A. Malignant lymphoma B. Malignant melanoma
   C. Ca lung   D. Hepatoblastoma

4. **Lymphoid pseudotumor of breast/differentiated from malignant lymphoma by :**
   A. Sharp border
   B. Presence of mature lymphocyter plasma cells and reticulum cells
   C. Proliferation of ductal cells
   D. All of the above

5. **The propensity of fibroadenomas to become malignant is :**
   A. Nil   B. Rare
   C. Sometimes D. Often

6. **Most common malignancy in AIDS :**
   A. Kaposi's sarcoma B. B cell lymphoma
   C. Leukemias   D. Burkitts Lymphoma

7. **Malignant tumors are at least —— times ——commoner than benign tumors in retroperito neum :**
   A. 2 more   B. 4 more
   C. 2 less   D. 4 less

8. **Commonest malignant tumor of retroperitoneum is :**
   A. Malignant lymphoma B. Liposarcoma
   C. Leiomyosarcoma   D. Pheochromocytoma

9. **Commonest neoplasm of retroperitoneal soft tissue is :**
   A. Liposarcoma B. Leiomyosarcoma
   C. Lymphoma   D. Pheochromocytoma

Ans.	1. A	2. A	3. D	4. D	5. A	6. A
	7. B	8. A	9. A			

10. **Paragangliomas may show production of :**
    A. ACTH   B. Catecholamines
    C. GH   D. ADH

11. **Mitotic counts of atleast ———— or more per HPF indicate a diagnosis of leiomyosarcoma :**
    A. 1   B. 3
    C. 5   D. 20

12. **"Orphan Annie cells" are seen in :**
    A. Struma ovari
    B. Retinoblastoma
    C. Papillary cell carcinoma of thyroid
    D. Melanoma of eye

13. **Chloroma is a tumor of :**
    A. Soft tissue   B. Bone
    C. Haemopoeitic cell   D. Ovary

14. **Breast cancer is predisposed by :**
    A. Increase in androgen
    B. Increase in oestrogen
    C. Decrease in oestrogen
    D. Decrease in androgen

15. **Ca thyroid with good prognosis :**
    A. Follicular   B. Lymphoma
    C. Papillary   D. All equal

16. **Which of the following is untrue of angiomyolipoma :**
    A. Locally invasive
    B. Doesn't metastasize
    C. Cerebral pulmonary and cutaneous hamoartamas of tuberous sclerosis may be associated
    D. Hematuria may occur

17. **Male 3 yrs. Abdominal mass. Rounded well circumscribed greyish white lesion 5 x 4 x 6 cms with rhabdomyoblasts and sheets of anaplastic cells adjacent kidney tissue is likely to be :**
    A. Hypernephroma   B. Wilm's tumour
    C. Hamartoma   D. Neuroblastoma

18. **Call-Exner bodies may be seen in all of the following except :**
    A. Gonadoblastoma of the ovary
    B. Arrhenoblastoma of the ovary
    C. Granulosa cell tumours of ovary
    D. Ripening follicles in infants

Ans.	10. B	11. C	12. C.	13. C	14. B	15. C
	16. A	17. B	18. B			

19. **Chemodectomas can occur in all of the following sites except :**
    A. Retroperitoneum   B. GIT
    C. Eyes   D. Lungs

20. .The common cause of death in choriocarcinoma is :
    A. Liver failure   B. Infection
    C. Haemorrhage   D. Local invasion

21. **Lacunar cells are characteristically seen in :**
    A. Lymphocyte predominant Hodgkin's disease
    B. Nodular scelrosis type of Hodgkin's disease
    C. Mixed cellularity type of Hodgkin's disease
    D. Lymphocyte depleted type Hodgkin's

22. **The incidence of which of the following cancers has increased in the past 4 decades :**
    A. Carcinoma of pancreas B.   Carcinoma of stomach
    C. Carcinoma of lung   D.   Carcinoma of colon
    E. a & c only

23. **Workers is vinyl chloride industry are known to develop :**
    A. Adenocarcinoma of the lung
    B. Angiosarcoma of the liver
    C. Polyposis of the colon
    D. Angiofibroma of the nose

24. **This is considered to be premalignant condition in the breast :**
    A. Pubertal hyperplasia   B.   Mammary dysplasia
    C. Plasma cell mastitis   D.   Galactocele

25. **Adenoidcystic carcinoma is a slow growing adenocarcinoma seen in all the following except :**
    A. Paranasal sinues   B.   Trachea
    C. Breast   D.   Small intestine

26. **Brooke's tumor is a tumor of :**
    A. Superficial dermal vessels
    B. Sweat glands
    C. Hair follicles
    D. Sebaceous glands

27. **Extranodal lymphomas are common in the :**
    A. Lung
    B. Gastro intestinal tract
    C. Male genital tract
    D. Central nervous system

Ans.	19. D	20. C	21. B	22. E	23. B	24. B
	25. D	26. C	27. B			

28. Which tumour is throught to arise from the chorionic   villi :
    A. Endodermal sinus tumour
    B. Choriocarcinoma
    C. Syncytioma
    D. All of the above

29. Burkitt's lymphoma is due to :
    A. Industrial dust   B. Bacteria
    C. Herpes group of virus D. Rickettsiae

30. The most usual mode of death in cancer patients is :
    A. Infections   B. Organ failure
    C. Infarction   D. Carcinomatosis
    E. Haemorrhage

31. Glomus tumour is :
    A. Lympagiosarcoma   B. Angiomyoneuroma
    C. Neurofibrolipoma   D. Painless

32. The commonest type of carcinoma breast is :
    A. Schirrhous   B. Papillary
    C. Follicular   D. Paget's disease

33. All are expansible secondaries are seen in :
    A. Renal cell carcinoma   B. Basal cell carcinoma
    C. Osteogenic sarcoma   D. Carcinoma prostate

34. The commonest benign soft tissue is :
    A. Lipoma   B. Leimyoma
    C. Hamartoma   D. Fibroma

35. Which of the following is genetically determined :
    A. Villous tumour   B. Adeno carcinoma
    C. Oat cell tumour   D. Carcinoma caecum

36. Term etal adenoma is used for :
    A. Hepatoma liver
    B. Fibroadenoma breast
    C. Follicular adenoma thyroid
    D. Craniopharyngioma

37. The commonest tumor of parotid is :
    A. Mucoepidermoid   B. Mixed parotid tumour
    C. Adenolymphoma   D. Squamous cell carcinoma

38. Rossette shaped arrangement of cells are seen in :
    A. Thecoma ovary   B. Ependymoma
    C. Neurofibroma   D. Lymphoma

39. Giant cells are least likely to be seen in :
    A. Osteosarcoma   B. Rhabdomyosarcoma
    C. Liposarcoma   D. Brenner's tumour

Ans.	28. D	29. C	30. A	31. B	32. A	33. A
	34. A	35. A	36. C	37. B	38. B	39. A

40. **About sarcoma true is :**
    A. Enucleation
    B. Histology predicts prognosis
    C. Spread to lymph nodes
    D. May be sensitive to radiotherapy

41. **Commonest malignancy in males in western countries is of :**
    A. Mouth   B. Lungs
    C. Larynx   D. Rectum

42. **Nasopharyngeal angiofibromas are most frequently seen in the :**
    A. I decade   B. II decade
    C. III decade   D. IV decade
    E. VI-VII decade

43. **Paget's disease is seen in :**
    A. Bone   B. Breast
    C. Vulva   D. All
    E. None

44. **Luke's classification in associated with :**
    A. Lymphoma   B. Hodgkin's disease
    C. Carcinoma cervix D. Carcinoma bladder

45. **Sarcoma metastasizes mainly through :**
    A. Blood   B. Lymphatic channels
    C. Infiltration   D. Along perineural sheath
    E. Any of the above

46. **Tumor can be easily diagnosed by :**
    A. Exfoliative cytology B. Endoscopy
    C. Histopathology   D. Tumor markers only
    E. All of the above

47. **Carcinomas especially likely to cause fever   include :**
    A. Hypernephroma   B. Carcinoma stomach
    C. Carcinoma pancreas D. All of these
    E. a + b

48. **Kulchitsky cells are seen in :**
    A. Adamantionoma   B. Wilm's tumour
    C. Hypernephroma   D. Argentiffinoma

49. **The following turmours in human beings are believed to be of viral origin except :**
    A. Hodgkin's disease
    B. Hepatic carcinoma
    C. Nasopharyngeal carcinoma
    D. Uterine cervical carcinoma

Ans.	40. B	41. B	42. B	43. 44. A	45. A	46. A
	47. D	48. D	49. A			

50. In which of the following carcinoma, metastasis disappears if primary is removed surgically :
   A. Colon   B. Kidney
   C. Melanoma   D. Lung
51. Commonest malignancy in children is :
   A. Lymphoma   B. Leukaemia
   C. Neuroblastoma   D. Wilm's tumour
52. Malignancies caused by viruses are :
   A. Nasopharyngeal carcinoma
   B. Burkitt's lymphoma
   C. Carcinoma cervix
   D. All of the above
53. The tumor formerly known as chloroma is better designated as
   A. Malignant lymphoma
   B. Monocytic leukemia
   C. Granulocytic sarcoma
   D. Multiple myeloma
   E. Tumor of plant cell origin
54. Ameloblastoma (Adamantinoma) is found in :
   A. Pituitary   B. Mandible
   C. Tibia   D. All of the above
55. Serum calcium level is increased in all except :
   A. Multiple myeloma
   B. Secondary carcinomatosis
   C. Myxedema
   D. Primary hyperparathyroidism
56. Vinyl chloride has been implicated in :
   A. Angiosarcoma of liver B. Angiofibroma of nose
   C. Hepatomas   D. Bladder cancer
57. Commonest carcinoma in elderly male is :
   A. Stomach   B. Lung
   C. Esophagus   D. Prostate
58. Cementifying fibromas are characterised by all of the following except :
   A. Sheets, bundles and whorls of fibrous connective tissue
   B. Spherites of cementum
   C. Numerous mitotic figures
   D. Islands of osteoid and bony spicules
59. Rarely metastasizes :
60. Frequently occurs in siblings

Ans.	50. B	51. B	52. D	53. C	54. D	55. C
	56. A	57. D	58. D	59. C	60. A	

61. Associated with alcoholism and smoking
62. Contains abundant lipid
63. Frequently spreads by invading vein :
    Match Questions 255-256
    A. Sq. cell carcinoma of skin
    B. Basal cell carcinoma of skin
    C. Both
    D. Neither
64. Predisposed to by chronic exposure to sunlight :
65. Rareley, if ever metastasizes :
66. The least common of the following types of breast neoplasm is :
    A. Indurating ductal carcinoma
    B. Infiltrating lobular carcinoma
    C. Cystosarcoma phylloides
    D. Mucinous carcinoma
    E. Medullary carcinoma
67. Non-capsulated benign tumour is :
    A. Fibroleiomyoma   B. Capillary haemangioma
    C. Rectal adenoma   D. All of the above
68. Rhabdomyosarcomas usually arise in children in :
    A. Thigh muscle   B. Heart muscle
    C. Vagina   D. Body of uterus
69. Carcinomas commonly metastasize to all of the following sites except :
    A. Skeletal muscle   B. Lymph nodes
    C. Kidney   D. Brain
70. Lipoma which becomes malignant is :
    A. Retroperitoneal   B. Subcutaneous
    C. Mediastinal   D. Subfascial
71. Tumour marker for a highly vascular tu-mour :
    A. Desmin   B. Keratin
    C. SA 200   D. None
72. Scirrhous carcinoma is a name given to :
    A. A carcinoma of breast with the lot of fibrous tissue in between tumour cells
    B. A carcinoma of breast which involves and puckers the skin
    C. A carcinoma of breast which is non infiltrating
    D. All of the above

Ans.	61. D	62. E	63. E	64. C	65. B	66. C
	67. D	68. C	69. A	70. A	71. C	72. A

73. The most rapidly sprading malignant tumours in the given examples is :
   A. Chorio carcinoma of uterus
   B. Carcinoma of breast
   C. Mucinous cyst adenocarcinoma of ovary
   D. None of the above

74. An encapuslated rubbery breast tumour is most likely a :
   A. Scirrhous Carcinoma   B. Midullary Carcinoma
   C. Colloid Carcinoma   D. Fibroadenoma

75. The poorest prognosis in terms of five year survival is offered by carcinoma of :
   A. Ovary   B. Prostate
   C. Cervix   D. Gall bladder
   E. Colon

76. Of the following, the five-year survival is highest in :
   A. Papillary adenocarcinoma of thyroid
   B. Follicular cardinoma of thyroid
   C. Undifferentitated cell carcinom of thyroid
   D. Transitional cell carcinoma of bladder
   E. Solid carcinoma of ovary

77. True about cancrum oris is following except :
   A. Follows chronic infections
   B. Treatment is excision and grafting
   C. Involves jaw
   D. Involves primarily cheek and lips

78. Type of carcinoma of breast occurring bilaterally :
   A. Lobular carcinoma
   B. Infiltrating intraductal carcinoma
   C. Scirrhous carcinoma
   D. Colloid carcinoma
   E. Medullary carcinoma

79. Klatskin tumor is :
   A. Carcinoma head of the pancreas
   B. Carcinoma located at the junction of hepatic ducts
   C. Carcinoma ampulla of Vater
   D. Carcinoma body of pancreas

80. Homer-Wright rosettes are seen in :
   A. Neuroblastoma   B. Astrocytoma
   C. Meningioma   D. Pinealoma

Ans.	73. A	74. D	75. D	76. A	77. C	78. A
	79. B	80. A				

81. Carcinosarcoma most commonly occurs in :
    A. Uterus   B. Liver
    C. Breast   D. Lungs
82. Least malignant potential is seen in :
    A. Juvenile polyp   B. Turcot syndrome
    C. Gardner syndrome   D. Familial polyposis
83. All of the following chromosomal disorders are associated with advanced maternal age except :
    A. Down's syndrome   B. Edward's syndrome
    C. Cri-du-chat syndrome D. Patau's syndrome
84. Direct-acting carcinogens include :
    A. Nitrosamines   B. Polycyclic hydrocarbons
    C. Alkylating agents   D. tocopherol
85. Stony hard painless lymphnode in left supraclavicular fossa, biopsy reveals Sq. cell carcinoma, disease is :
    A. Lung carcinoma   B. Ca stomach
    C. Ca Breast   D. Ca Pancreas
86. MALTOMA is associated with :
    A. Hodgkin's lymphoma
    B. NHL
    C. Burkitt's lymphoma
    D. H. Pylori gastric lymphoma
87. Paget's cell in breast Ca :
    A. Vacuolated cytoplasm
    B. Multinodular giant cell
    C. Eosinophilic cytoplasm
    D. Basophilic giant cell
88. "Biphasic pattern" on histology is seen in which tumor?
    A. Rhabdomyosarcoma   B. Synovial cell sarcoma
    C. Osteosarcoma   D. Neurofibroma
89. Which of the following is curable tumor ?
    A. Lymphoma
    B. Carcinoma cervix
    C. Papillary carcinoma thyroid
    D. Ewing's tumor
90. All of the following type of lymphoma are commonly seen in orbit except :
    A. Non-Hodgkin's lymphoma (NHL), mixed lymphocytic and histiocytic
    B. NHL, lymphocytic poorly differentiated
    C. Burkitt's lymphoma
    D. Hodgkin's lymphoma

Ans.	81. A	82. A	83. B	84. C	85. A	86. D
	87. B	88. D	89. C	90. D		

91. Biopsy from a mole on the foot shows cytologic Atypia of melanocytes and diffuse epidermal infiltration by Anaplastic cells, which are also present in the papillary and reticular dermis. The most likely diagnosis is?
    - A. Melanoma, Clark level IV
    - B. Congenital melanocytic nevus
    - C. Dysplastic nevus
    - D. Melanoma, Clark level III

92. Primary malignant neoplasms are rare in the :
    - A. Oesophagus   B. Stomach
    - C. Small bowel   D. Large bowel

93. Metastasis to bone is not a feature of :
    - A. Ca rectum   B. Renal cell carcinoma
    - C. Ca thyroid   D. Ca breast

94. Proven tumour specific antigen is for all of the following except :
    - A. Gastric carcinoma   B. Burkitt's lymphoma
    - C. Carcimoma of breast   D. Neuroblastoma
    - E. Carcinoma colon

95. The most highly radioresistant tumour, of the following   is :
    - A. Squamous cell carcinoma
    - B. Fibrosarcoma
    - C. Lymphosarcoma
    - D. Embryonal.carcinoma

96. Secondaries not responding to chemotherapy are of :
    - A. Bone   B. Brain
    - C. Lung   D. Lymphatics

97. Solid tumor which responds best to 5-FU is of :
    - A. Pancreas   B. Thyroid
    - C. Colon   D. Lung

98. Surgical treatment can cure following tumours except :
    - A. Fibrosarcoma   B. Insulinoma
    - C. Glucagonoma   D. Appendicular carcinoid
    - E. Phaeochromocytoma

99. Earliest tumour to appear after birth is :
    - A. Sternomastoid tumour B. Cystic hygroma
    - C. Branchial cyst   D. Lymphoma

100. Chemotherapy is not indicated in :
    - A. Teratoma testis   B. Ca breast
    - C. Malignant melanoma D. Adenocarcinoma colon

Ans.	91. C	92. C	93. A	94. A	95. B	96. A
	97. A	98. A	99. B	100. C		

101. **Tamoxifen may be used in :**
    A. Ca breast　　　　　　B.　Ca prostate
    C. Ca thyroid　　　　　　D.　Ca pancreas

102. **Chemotherapy is not yet effective in :**
    A. Pancreatic Ca
    B. Choriocarcinoma of testis
    C. Testicular seminoma
    D. Vulval Ca

103. **Match List I with List II and select the correct answer using the codes given below the lists :**

List I		List II
A. Hodgkin's disease	1.	Adriamycin, Mitomycin, 5-fluoro-uracil
B. Breast carcinoma	2.	Cyclophosphamide, Methotrexate, 5-fluorouracil
C. Cancer buccal mucosa	3.	Cyclophosphamide, Oncovin, Procarbazine, Prednisolone
D. Cancer stomach	4.	Cisplatinum, 5- fluorouracil

    Codes :

	A	B	C	D
A.	3	2	1	4
B.	2	3	1	4
C.	3	2	4	1
D.	3	2	1	4

104. **Gleasen's staging is done in :**
    A. Ca prostate　　　　　　B.　Ca Pancreas
    C. CA kidney　　　　　　　D.　Ca Cx

105. **Match List I (Primary malignancies) with List II (Most common site of metastasis and select the correct answer :**

List I		List II
A. Prostatic carcinoma	1.	Left supraclavicular lymph nodes
B. Seminoma testis	2.	Lungs
C. Carcinoma stomach	3.	Lumbar vertebrae
D. Choriocarcinoma	4.	Paraortic lymph nodes

	A	B	C	D
A.	3	4	2	1
B.	4	3	1	2
C.	4	3	2	1
D.	3	4	1	2

Ans.　101. A　　　102. B　　　103. C　　　104. A　　　105. D

106. A 20 year old male presented with chronic constipation, headache and palpitations. On examination he had marfanoid habitus, neuromas of tongue, medullated corneal nerve fibres and a nodule of 2 ´ 2 cms size in the left lobe of thyroid gland. This patient is a case of ?
  A. Sporadic medullary carcinoma of thyroid
  B. Familial medullary carcinoma of thyroid
  C. MEN IIA
  D. MEN IIB

Ans.   106. D

RECENT QUESTIONS

1. Now the diagnosis of Barret's esophagus is made by demonstration of columnar mucosa which on hitopathology shows :   AIIMS 2012
   A. Intestinal metaplasia
   B. Intestinal dysplasia
   C. Columnar metaplasia
   D. Squamous dysplasia

2. Jaw cyst which is most prone to malignancy is :   AIIMS 2011, 2012
   A. Dental cyst   B. Dentigerous cyst
   C. Odontogenic keratocyst D. Radicular cyst

3. Second primary malginancy of head and neck is commonly associated with which of the following :   AIIMS 2012
   A. Oral cavity   B. Hypopharynx
   C. Larynx   D. Paranasal sinuses

4. The most characteristic histological feature of basal cell carcinoma is :
                                                    AI 2012; AIIMS 2012
   A. Foamy cells   B. Nuclear palisading
   C. Keratin pearls   D Psammoma bodies

5. In a patient with breast carcinoma stage tub as per TNM classification is defined by all of the following except ;   AIIMS 2006, 2012
   A. Nipple retraction
   B. Dermal edema
   C. Skin ulceration overtumor
   D. Sattellite lesions in involved breast

6. Cancer management in which of the following malignancies has dramatically increasd the survival :   AIIMS 2012
   A. Esophagus carcinoma   B. Glioblastoma multiforme
   C. ALL in children   D. Cholangiocarcinoma

7. A 35 year-old woman was found to have Ca cervix, FIGO stage 2-3, locally advanced what would be management :   AIIMS 2012
   A. Surgery plus chemotherapy
   B. Radiotherapy plus chemotherapy
   C. Chemotherapy
   D. Radiotherapy plus HPV vaccine

Ans.	1. A	2. C	3. A	4. B	5. A	6. C
	7. B					

8. A patient with known mutation in the 'Rb gene' is disease free from retinoblastoma. The patient is at highest risk of developing which of the following malignancies: **AI 2010 ; AIIMS 2012**
    A. Renal cell carcinoma   B. Osteosarcoma
    C. Pinealoblastoma   D. Chondroblastoma

9. Chromophobe variant of Renal cell carcinoma is associated with:
    AI 2010
    A. VHL gene mutations
    B. Trisomy of 7 and 17 (+7, +17)
    C. 3 p deletions (3p-)
    D. Monosomy of 1 and Y (-1,-Y)

10. Which of the following tests is not used for detection of specific aneuploidy: **AI 2007; 2010**
    A. FISH   B. RT-PCR
    C. QP-PCR   D. Microarray

11. An example of tumor suppressor gene is: **AIIMS 2005**
    A. Myc   B. fos
    C. ras   D. Rb

12. Most chemoresistant tumours among the following is: **AIIMS 2006**
    A. Synovial sarcoma
    B. Osteosarcoma
    C. Malignant fibrous histiocytoma
    D. Embryonal rhabdomyosarcoma

13. Least risk of Ca breast is seen is: **AIIMS 2006**
    A. BRCA 1   B. BRCA2
    C. Li-Fraumeni syndrome   D. Ataxia telangiectasia

14. Which one of the following is not used as a tumour marker in testicular tumours: **AP 2005**
    A. AFP   B. LDH   .
    C. HCG   D. CEA

15. Biphasic pattern on histology is seen in which tumour: **Delhi 2010**
    A. Rhabdomyosarcoma
    B. Synovial cell sarcoma
    C. Osteosarcoma
    D. Neurofibroma

16. Mantle cell lymphomas are positive for all of the following except:
    A. CD23   B. CD5
    C. CD20   D. Cyclic D1

Ans.	8. B	9. D	10. D	11. D	12. C	13. D
	14. D	15. B	16. A			

17. **False about the malignant ulcer of stomach is:**   **Delhi 2010**
    A. The mucosal folds do not reach the edge of the ulcer
    B. Mucosal folds are thickened and fused
    C. Ulcer crator is eccentric
    D. Margins of the ulcer are overhanging

18. **Findings of multiple myeloma in kidney are all except:**

    Delhi 2010; 2011

    A. Tubular casts   B. Amyloidosis
    C. Wire loop lesions   D. Renal tubular necrosis

19. **Pseudolymphoma is manifestation of :**   **Delhi 2010**
    A. Phenytoin   B. Sodium valproate
    C. Carbamazepine   D. Phenobarbitone

20. **Neoadjuvant chemotherapy is used in all except:**   **Delhi 2010; 2011**
    A. Esophageal Ca   B. Breast Ca
    C. Thyroid Ca   D. Long non-small cell Ca

21. **All of the following hereditary conditions predispose to CNS tumors except:**   **Delhi 2008; 2010**
    A. Neurofibromatosis 1 and 2
    B. Tuberous sclerosis
    C. von Hippel Lindau syndrome
    D. Xeroderma pigmentosum

22. **A 60-year old male was diagnosed with carcinoma right lung. On CECT chest there was tumour of 5× 5 cm in upper lobe and another 2×2 cm size tumour nodule in middle lobe. The primary modality of treatment is:**

    Delhi 2010

    A. Radiotherapy   B. Chemotherapy
    C. Surgery   D. Supportive treatment

23. **All the following increase risk for cholangiocarcinoma except:**

    Delhi 2010

    A. Ulcerative colitis
    B. Gall stones in CBD
    C. Sclerosing cholangitis
    D. Chlonorchis sinensis

24. **Which is not true of carcinoma tongue:**   **Delhi 2010**
    A. Lateral border is involved
    B. Cervical lymph node involvement
    C. Commonly adenocarcinoma
    D. Tobacco chewing is a risk factor

Ans.	17. D	18. C	19. A	20. C	21. D	22. C
	23. B	24. C				

25. Carcinoma of fundus of uterus can spread to all the following lymph nodes except: Delhi 2010
    A. Inguinal   B. Obturator
    C. Intenal iliac   D. Para-aortic

26. In patients with breast cancer, chest wall involvement means involvement of any one of the following structures except: Delhi 2010
    A. Serratus anterior
    B. Pectoralis Major·
    C. Intercostal Mucles
    D. Ribs

27. The colposcopic feature suggestive of malignancy are all except:
                                                                      Delhi 2010
    A. Condyloma   B. Vascular atypia
    C. Punctuation   D. White epithelium

28. A patient with carcinoma cervix who has completed radiotherapy comes with uraemia. The most common cause is: Delhi 2010
    A. Bilateral ureter invasion
    B. Radiation nephritis
    C. Ureteric stenosis due to radiation
    D. Unconnected causes

29. Increased risk of cancer is seen in :   Delhi 2009
    A. Fibroadenoma of breast
    B. Bronchial asthma
    C. Chronic ulcerative colitis
    D. Leiomyomas of the uterus

30. A chronic alcoholic has an elevated serum alpha fetoprotein levels. Which of the following neoplasms is most likley: Delhi 2009
    A. Prostatic adenocarcinoma
    B. Multiple myeloma
    C. Hepatocellular carcinoma
    D. Glioblastoma multiforme

31. Antitumor activity is shown by all except: Delhi 2009
    A. Cytotoxic T lymphocytes
    B. Natural killer cells
    C. Basophils
    D. Macrophages

Ans.	25. B	26. B	27. A	28. A	29. C	30. C
	31. C					

32.   In the testis, intratubular germ cell neoplasia is seen in all, except:

       Delhi 2009

       A. Seminomas
       B. Spermatocytic seminoma
       C. Yolk sac tumor of testis
       D. Enbryonal carcinoma

33.   The most common malignancy found in Marjolin's ulcer is: **Delhi 2009**
       A. Basal cell carcinoma
       B. Squamous cell carcinoma
       C. Malignant fibrous histiocytoma
       D. Neutrophic malignant melanoma

34.   The following bone tumour may cause dural deposits without causing bony changes: **Delhi 2009**
       A. Hodgkin's lymphoma   B. Multiple myeloma
       C. Secondaries   D. Fibrous dysplasia

35.   The most important prognostic factor in carcinoma breast is:

       Delhi 2009

       A. Size of tumour
       B. Skin involvement
       C. Involvement of muscles
       D   Axillary gland involvement

36.   Commonest benign tumour of the esophagus: **Delhi 2009**
       A. Leiomyoma   B. Papilloma
       C. Adenoma   D. Hemangioma

37.   Solitary nodule lung cannot be: **Delhi 2009**
       A. Tuberculoma
       B. Neurofibroma
       C. Bronchogenic carcinoma
       D. Lymphoma

38.   A 40 years old female patient presented with recurrent headaches. MRI showed extra axial, dural based and enhancing lesion. The most likely diagnosis is: **Delhi 2009**
       A. Meningioma   B. Glioma
       C. Schwanoma   D. Pituitary adenoma

39.   Radioactive phosphorus is used in the treatment of: **Delhi 2009**

       A. Polycythemia
       B. Thyroid metastasis
       C. Multiple myeloma
       D. Embryonal cell carcinoma

Ans.	32. B	33. B	34. A	35. D	36. A	37. B
	38. A	39. A				

40. Most radio dense substance is: Delhi 2009
   A. Fluid
   B. Soft tissue
   C. Brain
   D. Bone

41. The tissue most resistant to radioactivity is: Delhi 2010
   A. Rectum
   B. Colon
   C. Cervix
   D. Vagina

42. Hyperfractionation radiotherapy is used in the management of:
   Delhi 2009
   A. Lung cancer
   B. Breast cancer
   C. Seminoma
   D. Ovarian cancer

43. Chemosensitive tumors are all, except: Delhi 2009
   A. Carcinoma cervix
   B. Ewing's sarcoma
   C. Osteosarcoma
   D. Ca breast

44. Which of the following is not correct about fibrolamellar variant of Hepatocellular carcinoma: Delhi 2009
   A. Occurs in young males and females
   B. Hepatitis B virus is an important risk factor
   C. Often has a better prognosis
   D. Is a hard scirrhous tumour

45. Hybridoma refers to: Delhi 2009
   A. Collision tumor
   B. A tumor of brown fat
   C. A hamartoma
   D. A technnique for rating monoclonal antibodies

46. Which of the following liver tumors always merit surgery? Delhi 2009
   A. Hemangioma
   B. Hepatic adenoma
   C. Focal nodular hyperplasia
   D. Peliosis hepatic

47. Rare histological variants of carcinoma breast with better prognosis include all except: Delhi 2009
   A. Colloid carcinoma
   B. Medullary carcinoma
   C. Inflammatory carcinoma
   D. Tubular carcinoma

48. The risk of sarcoma developing in a fibroid uterus is approximately:
   Delhi 2009
   A. <1%
   B. 10%
   C. 30%
   D. 50%

Ans.	40. B	41. D	42. A	43. A	44. B	45. A
	46. B	47. C	48. A			

49. The most characteristic presentation of fallopian tube carcinoma is:

Delhi 2009

- A. Mass abdomen
- B. Bleeding per vaginum
- C. Excessive watery discharge per vaginus
- D. Pain abdomen

50. Carcinoma cervix originates in the: Delhi 2009
- A. Columnar epithelium   B. Squamous epithelium
- C. Transformation zone   D. Uterine isthmus

51. An ovarian neoplasm in a 14-year old girl is most likely to be:

Delhi 2009

- A. Germ cell tumor
- B. Epithelial tumour
- C Sertolic Leydig cell tumor
- D. Granulosa cell tumor

52. The incidence of bilaterality in a dermoid cyst is approximately:

Delhi 2009

- A. 10%   B. 30%
- C. 50%   D. 70%

53. Most radio-sensitive stage is: Delhi 2009
- A. S-phase   B. G_2
- C. G_1 D. G_2M

54. A young adolesant male presents with dyspnea and is observed to have a mediastinal mass. Which of the following lymphomas is the most likely cause: Delhi 2009
- A. Diffuse large B cell lymphoma
- B. B cell rich T cell lymphoma
- C. Mediastinal rich B cell lymphoma
- D. Precursor T cell ALL

55. All of the following statements about carcinoid tumors are true, except:
- A. It is the most common malignant tumor of the small intestine
- B. Extensive involvement of small intestine is associated with higher probability of lung metastasis
- C. 5 year survival for carcinoid tumors is > 60%
- D. Appendiceal carcinoids are more common in females

Ans.	49. C	50. C	51. A	52. A	53. D	54. D
	55. A					

56. Most common cause of isolated splenic metastasis is: AI 2012
    - A. Ca pancreas   B   Ca stomach
    - C. Ca ovary   D. Ca cervix

57. A 55-year-old lady presents with abdominal distension, bleeding, pelvic pain and respiratory distress. Clinically examination reveals features of ascitis and CA-125 levels are elevated. This most likely diagnosis:
        AI 2012
    - A. Ca-ovary   B. Ca-cervix
    - C. Ca-Lung   D. Lymphoma

58. Tumor arising from olfactory nasal mucosa is: AI 2012
    - A. Nasal glioma
    - B. Adenoid cystic carcinoma
    - C. Nasopharyngeal carcinoma
    - D. Esthesioneuroblastoma

59. Which of the following liver metastasis appear hypo-echoic on ultrasonography: AI 2012
    - A. Breast cancer   B. Colon cancer
    - C. Renal carcinoma   D. Mucinous adenocarcinoma

60. Extra axial Intracranial lesion showing contrast enhancement on MRI is suggestive of: AI 2012
    - A. Meningioma   B. Ependymoma
    - C. Arachnoid cyst   D. Astrocytoma

Ans.   56. C   57. A   58. D   59. A   60. A

Review Paper
(Based on Latest MCQs)

1. On immunohistochemistry, classical Hodgkin's lymphoma Reed Sternberg cells are likely to be
   A. CD15(-), CD 30(+),CD45(-)   B. CD15(+), CD 30(+),CD45(+)
   C. CD15(+), CD 30(+),CD45(-)   D. CD15(-), CD 30(+),CD45(+)
2. Involvement of which of the following organ is likely to be associated with poor outcome in primary amyloidosis
   A. cardiac   B. renal
   C. skin   D. liver
3. Which one of the following cancers is usually associated with a moderate to high uptake of ^{18}F-fluorodeoxyglucose (18 FFDG)?
   A. Bladder   B. Colorectal
   C. Thyroid   D. Testicular
4. Cytotoxic T cells (CTL) are capable of recognizing all EXCEPT:
   A. Peptide antigens associated with major histocompatibility complex (MHC) molecules
   B. Cytoplasmic antigens
   C. Nuclear antigens
   D. None of the above
5. Previous clinical studies with cancer vaccines have:
   A. Clearly demonstrated induction of tumor-specific immune response
   B. Repeatedly demonstrated clinical response to large tumor burden
   C. Not clearly demonstrated induction of tumor-specific immune response
   D. Not been performed to date
6. Which of the following chemotherapy drug is likely to be toxic to gonads?

Ans.   1 C   2 A   3 B   4 D   5 C   6 D

A. Adriamycin   B. Vinblastine
C. Paclitaxel   D. Procarbazine

7. For allogenic hemopoietic stem cell transplantation in children with hemoglobinopathies. Presently best source of stem cells is:
   A. Bone marrow
   B. Umbilical cord
   C. Peripheral blood
   D. Bone marrow + peripheral blood

8. The presence of which marker is a significant poor prognosis variable for patients with breast cancer:
   A. CEA.   B. C-erb B-2.
   C. AFP.   D. RB-1

9. Which of the following is less likely to be associated with Gallbladder cancer?
   A. Obesity   B. Use of tobacco and alcohol
   C. Aflatoxins   D. Past history of enteric fever

10. Patients that have acquired immunodeficiency syndrome are at increased risk for which of the following neoplasms?
    A. Colorectal cancer   B. Meningioma
    C. Kaposi's sarcoma   D. Hepatocellular carcinoma

11. Which of the following is NOT among the uses of PET imaging in the management of cervical cancer?
    A. Initial diagnosis   B. Staging
    C. Treatment planning   D. Assessment of prognosis

12. Which of the following targeted agents is NOT a tyrosine kinase inhibitor that influences the human epidermal growth factor receptor (HER) family signaling pathway by binding to the intracellular domain of the receptors?
    A. Gefitinib (HER1 inhibitor)
    B. Erlotinib (HER1 inhibitor)
    C. Trastuzumab (HER2 inhibitor)
    D. Lapatinib (HER1/HER2 inhibitor)

13. A 57-year-old, obese white man has symptoms of chronic gastroesophageal reflux disease (GERD). Endoscopic evaluation reveals evidence of Barrett's esophagus with high-grade dysplasia. What is the recommended management for this disease?
    A. Repeated endoscopy in 3-5 years
    B. Annual endoscopy

C. Mucosal resection or endoscopic ablation therapies
D. None of the above

14. Rituximab in combination with CHOP (R-CHOP) was approved in 2006 by the FDA for treatment of diffuse large B-cell lymphoma (DLBCL). The addition of rituximab to standard chemotherapy has been shown to benefit the following patient population EXCEPT?
    A. Older patients
    B. Low-risk International Prognostic Index (IPI) patients
    C. High-risk IPI patients
    D. None of the above

15. The immunomodulating monoclonal antibody alemtuzumab is associated with which infectious complication EXCEPT?
    A. PCP   B. Mycobacterial infection
    C. CMV   D. Neurocysticercosis

16. Prostate-specific antigen (PSA) testing and digital rectal examination (DRE) for prostate cancer screening meet all of the following criteria for an effective screening tool EXCEPT:
    A. Prostate cancer is prevalent and serious enough to warrant screening
    B. Early, presymptomatic disease is detected by the screening test
    C. Evidence shows that early discovery of the disease reduces morbidity and/or mortality
    D. None of the above

17. A new marker that has possible utility in the management of patients with non–small-cell lung cancer (NSCLC) is:
    A. Calcitonin   B. Neuron-specific enolase
    C. CYFRA 21-1   D. Chromogranin A

18. A number of clinical factors have been noted to decrease sensitivity of tumors to the effects of ionizing radiation. Which of the following is most important in this regard?
    A. Increased tissue vascularity   B. High tumor mitotic rate
    C. Tissue hypoxia   D. Subcutaneous tumor location

19. Hemophilia B has been treated in a pre-clinical model by gene transfer for which deficient clotting factor?
    A. Factor II   B. Factor VII
    C. Factor IX   D. Factor X

20. Antidepressants have been shown to be effective for the treatment of hot flashes related to hormonal therapies for breast cancer. However, some may inhibit the enzyme CYP2D6, which converts tamoxifen to

its active form and thus may interfere with tamoxifen activity. Which of the following antidepressants inhibits CYP2D6 to the greatest degree?

A. Vilazodone
B. Sertraline
C. Paroxetine
D. Venlafaxine

21. All of the following are known to be strong risk factors for gastric cancer EXCEPT:

A. Helicobacter pylori infection
B. Smoking
C. Alcohol abuse
D. Previous gastric surgery

22. "Triple-negative" breast cancer has been defined by modern genomic techniques as which distinct breast tumor subset?

A. Luminal A
B. Luminal B
C. Basal-like
D. "Normal"-like

23. Which of the following viruses is/are considered to be neurotropic?

A. Adenovirus
B. Herpes simplex virus
C. Retrovirus
D. Adeno-associated virus

24. Which of the following statement relating to cystic fibrosis is/are correct?

A. Cystic fibrosis is inherited as an X chromosome-linked recessive trait
B. Cystic fibrosis is caused by a defective chloride channel
C. Cystic fibrosis is caused by defective acetylcholine receptors
D. Cystic fibrosis is inherited as an autosomal dominant trait

25. What is the best treatment approach for aggressive nonmelanoma skin cancer (NMSC) when disfigurement or functional impairment is a risk?

A. Mohs' micrographic surgery
B. Radiation therapy
C. Imiquimod
D. Photodynamic therapy

26. What percentage of all breast cancer cases is related to genetic susceptibility?

A. 10
B. 25
C. 37
D. 45

27. Temozolomide has emerged as an agent that is active against:

A. Multiple sclerosis
B. Myasthenia gravis
C. Glioblastoma multiforme
D. Endometrial carcinoma

28. Tyrosine kinase inhibitors include following EXCEPT:

A. Gefitinib
B. Erlotinib
C. Trastuzumab
D. Lapatinib

Ans.   21 C   22 C   23 B   24 B   25 A   26 B   27 C   28 C

29. A 73-year-old woman presents with iron deficiency anemia. She is found to have a right-sided colon cancer. Staging investigations are negative. She undergoes right hemicolectomy. There are no unexpected findings at surgery. The pathology report describes a low-grade adenocarcinoma involving the muscularis propria, but not beyond. Fourteen lymph nodes are negative for cancer. What is the TNM classification and overall stage of her cancer?
    A. T2N0M0, Stage I   B. T2N0M0, Stage II
    C. T2N0M1, Stage I   D. T2N0M1, Stage II

30. Spontaneous regression is a well-documented phenomenon in some advanced cancers. The cancers in which spontaneous regression has been reported include following EXCEPT:
    A. Renal carcinoma   B. Melanoma
    C. Low grade lymphoma   D. Meningioma

31. Sipuleucel-T is used in:
    A. Ca colon   B. Hepatic cell carcinoma
    C. Carcinoid   D. Prostate cancer

32. Ipilimumab is used in:
    A. Basal cell carcinoma B. Retinoblastoma
    C. Melanoma   D. Renal cell carcinoma

33. Although, radical surgery can be very effective in managing the primary tumour in many cancers, it can lead to impaired quality of life through loss of specific organ function. The cancer for which surgery can be replaced by radiotherapy (with or without systemic therapy) to allow organ preservation without compromising survival.
    A. Renal cell carcinoma B. Melanoma
    C. Laryngeal cancer   D. Osteosarcoma

34. A 42-year-old man with acromegaly had a MR scan of brain, which showed suprasellar extension of his tumour. His visual fields were assessed prior to surgery. What is the earliest visual field defect?
    A. Lower nasal quadrantanopia
    B. Lower temporal quadrantanopia
    C. Upper nasal quadrantanopia
    D. Upper temporal quadrantanopia

35. A 67-year-old man with myelofibrosis was referred for splenic irradiation for massive splenomegaly extending 18 cm below the left costal margin. He lived 62 miles from the radiotherapy centre. It was planned to treat him with 8 MV photons using a pair of parallel opposed

---

Ans. 29 A   30 D   31 D   32 C   33 C   34 D   35 A

fields. What is the most appropriate dose, fractionation and time schedule for his radiotherapy?

A. 16 Gy, eight weekly fractions over 7 weeks
B. 20 Gy, ten daily fractions, 14 days
C. 25 Gy, five fractions (alternate days), 12 days
D. 45 Gy, 25 daily fractions, 35 days

36. A 63-year-old woman was brought to the chemotherapy department distressed and complaining of a "blocked throat". The symptoms had started 20 minutes earlier when she was drinking a gin and tonic. She had lung metastases from colorectal cancer and had received her third cycle of oxaliplatin and 5-fluorouracil chemotherapy ten days earlier. On examination, her temperature was 36.9°C, respiratory rate was 22 breaths per minute, pulse was 80 bpm and blood pressure was 125/85 mmHg. There were no abnormal chest signs. Chest x-ray showed lung metastases. Her neutrophil count was 0.5 x 109/L (1.5-7.0). What is the most appropriate management?

A. Anticoagulation
B. Glyceryl trinitrate spray
C. High dose steroids
D. No active treatment

37. A 62-year-old woman presented with a two month history of abdominal pain and distension. Ultrasound showed a 3-cm liver metastasis and ascites. Her CA125 was 500 U/ml(<35); CEA was 25 µg/L (<10). Liver biopsy showed adenocarcinoma with the immunoprofile: CK7 +ve, CK20 –ve and TTF1 +ve. What is the most likely primary site?

A. Breast
B. Colon
C. Lung
D. Ovary
E. Thyroid

38. A 64-year-old man presented with dysphagia. Endoscopy showed a 6-cm adenocarcinoma of the lower third of the oesophagus. Endoscopic ultrasound showed a 2-cm para-oesophageal node. PET-CT scan showed no evidence of metastatic disease. What is the most appropriate treatment?

A. Neoadjuvant chemotherapy followed by surgery
B. Palliative chemotherapy
C. Pre-operative radiotherapy followed by surgery
D. Radical chemoradiotherapy

39. A 61-year-old man with a remote history of tobacco use presents with hematuria. He undergoes a transurethral resection (TUR), which reveals T1 superficial bladder cancer. What is his risk for bladder cancer recurrence in the next 5 years without further therapy?

Ans. **36 D** **37 C** **38 A** **39 D**

A. 10%   B. 30%

C. 50%   D. 70%

40. Treatment options for stage I nonseminomatous germ cell tumor (NSGCT) include all of the following, EXCEPT:

A. Surveillance or "watchful waiting"

B. Retroperitoneal lymph node dissection (RPLND)

C. Adjuvant chemotherapy

D. High-dose chemotherapy

41. The primary treatment for locoregionally advanced head and neck cancer consists of:

A. Surgery   B. Radiation therapy

C. Chemoradiation therapy   D. All of the above

42. Episodic acute overexposure to ultraviolet (UV) radiation (i.e., sunburn) is an important risk factor for following type of skin cancer EXCEPT:

A. Squamous cell carcinoma   B. Basal cell carcinoma

C. Melanoma   D. None of the above

43. Risk factors for anthracycline-induced cardiomyopathy include following EXCEPT:

A. Hypertension

B. Simultaneous administration with other neoplastic agents

C. Poor nutritional status

D. None of the above

44. What is the 5-year survival rate for patients who undergo curative hepatic resection of colorectal liver metastases?

A. < 5%   B. 10% to 20%

C. 30% to 40%   D. > 60%

45. Which characteristic is least likely for never-smokers who develop non-small cell lung cancer (NSCLC), compared with smokers who develop NSCLC?

A. Young   B. Female

C. Better survival rate   D. Worse survival rate

46. A 34-year-old woman presented with a 4-cm moderately differentiated adenocarcinoma of the anorectal junction. MR scan showed that the tumour has penetrated into the muscularis propria. There were no visible perirectal lymph nodes. What is the most appropriate management?

A. Abdominoperineal resection

B. Anterior resection

C. Pre-operative long-course chemoradiation and anterior resection

---

Ans.   **40 D**   **41 C**   **42 A**   **43 D**   **44 C**   **45 D**   **46 A**

    D. Pre-operative short-course radiotherapy and abdominoperineal resection

47. An 85-year-old woman presented with a 2 cm x 2 cm squamous cell carcinoma of the posterior auricular fold. It was 0.75- cm thick. What is the most appropriate treatment?
    A. 6 MeV electrons with 0.5 cm bolus, giving 55 Gy in 20 fractions over 4 weeks
    B. 12 MeV electrons with 0.5 cm bolus, giving 55 Gy in 20 fractions over 4 weeks
    C. Pinnectomy
    D. Wide excision plus grafting and radical neck dissection

48. A 68-year-old man had a 2-year history of right-sided hearing loss and balance problems. An MR scan of brain demonstrated a right cerebopontine angle enhancing tumour with a cystic component, consistent with an eighth nerve schwannoma. An axial slice is shown below. What is the most appropriate management?
    A. Observation with repeat MR scan of brain in 12 months
    B. Surgical resection
    C. Fractionated Stereotactic radiotherapy
    D. Stereotactic radiosurgery

49. Which of the following is universally considered to be the standard of care for resected pancreatic adenocarcinoma?
    A. Chemoradiation
    B. Chemoradiation plus chemotherapy
    C. 5-fluorouracil (5-FU)
    D. None of the above

50. Which of the following short-acting opioids used for breakthrough cancer-related pain has the most rapid onset of action?
    A. Morphine   B. Oxycodone
    C. Methadone   D. Transmucosal fentanyl

51. Which of the following variables best predicts prognosis for patients with a recent diagnosis of cutaneous melanoma and no clinical evidence of metastatic disease?
    A. Breslow thickness   B. Clark's level
    C. Ulceration   D. Gender

52. Bladder cancer is the fourth most common cancer in men and the eighth most common in women. As with many other diseases, the earlier that bladder cancer is diagnosed, the better the patient's long-term prognosis.

Ans.   **47 A**   **48 B**   **49 D**   **50 D**   **51 A**   **52 D**

What is the best screening test for bladder cancer?
A. Urine dipstick test
B. Urine cytology
C. Cystoscopy
D. No screening test is useful for universal screening

53. A 67-year-old man presented with frank haematuria. His past medical history included insulin-dependent diabetes for 10 years and coronary artery bypass surgery 2 years earlier. His WHO performance status was 1. Cystoscopy showed a 5-cm sessile tumour at the dome of the bladder. The bladder mucosa looked inflamed. Biopsy showed moderately differentiated transitional cell carcinoma invading superficial muscle. There was extensive carcinoma *in situ*. CT scan of chest and abdomen showed no pelvic or para-aortic lymphadenopathy and chest was normal. What is the most appropriate treatment for his bladder tumour?
A. Intravesical BCG weekly for 6 weeks
B. Intravesical mitomycin C weekly for 6 weeks
C. Palliative radiotherapy
D. Radical cystectomy

54. A 62-year-old man presented with a 3-day history of fever and purulent cough. His WHO performance status was: Chest X-ray showed a lesion in the left upper zone. His respiratory symptoms resolved completely after a course of antibiotics. There were no abnormal physical signs. Further investigations suggested a T2 N0 M0 squamous cell carcinoma involving the left main bronchus. Spirometry showed a FEV1 of 1.1 litres and a FVC of 1.9 litres. What is the most appropriate management?
A. high-dose palliative radiotherapy
B. left pneumonectomy
C. platinum-based chemotherapy
D. radical radiotherapy

55. What is a contraindication to the use of bevacizumab in patients with metastatic non-small-cell lung cancer (NSCLC)?
A. Previous hemoptysis   B. Brain metastases
C. Anticoagulation   D. All of the above

56. Which of the following chemopreventive agents has been shown to lower prostate cancer occurrence?
A. Finasteride   B. Lycopene
C. Selenium   D. All of the above

Ans.   53 D   54 D   55 D   56 A